ACKNOWLEDGEMENTS AND THANK YOU'S

I've had an overwhelming amount of support along the way in both my writing journey as well as my personal one. As rewarding as it is, writing can be an isolating and solitary endeavor. I'm immensely grateful for those who have made this process feel like anything but lonely. I'm surrounded by amazing people day in and day out who inspire me, teach me, advise me and keep me accountable. First and foremost, I want to thank my amazing children Jake and Emma. Thank you for always being my "why". You are my most profound reason for inspiring change in others and for striving to become a better human. You are the heartbeat behind this book. To my mom, Diane Dupuis Lazare. There has never been a time in my life where I didn't feel 100% supported by you. Thank you for loving me unconditionally. To my clients and friends. You are my family. You've been instrumental in this process and helped me grow as a coach and as a person. Because of you I have a calling and not a job. I'm forever indebted to you. To my colleagues: I've learned so much and continue to learn from you all every day. My dear friend and mentor Brian Grasso — thank you for shaping my direction in so many positive ways. You have given me so much of your wisdom and have taught me how to create change. Tom Venuto - I've learned so much from you over the years and I cannot thank you enough for taking a chance on my writing years ago. Sumi Singh: My cover model and amazing support over the years. Andréia: Thank you for your unwavering encouragement and for championing my crazy ideas. To my Lean Minded family: I wouldn't be here without you. I'm so honored that you follow my work and invest your time reading what I have to say. Thank you for your constant inspiration to create more content and continue to change lives.

With love, gratitude hugs and high 5's,
Mike

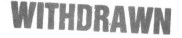

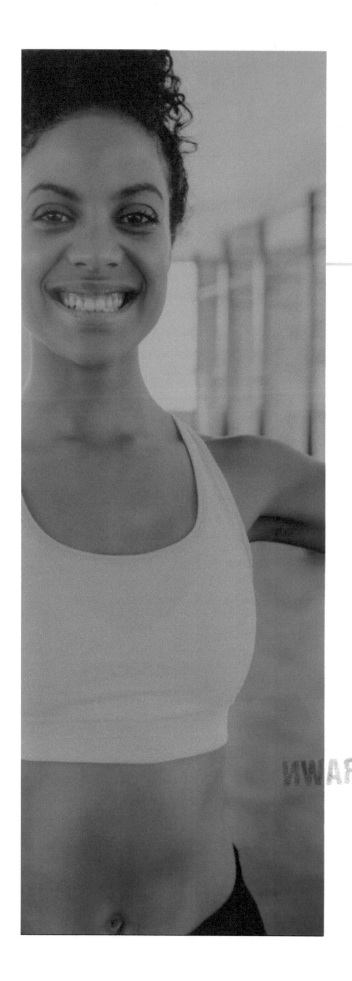

TABLE OF CONTENTS

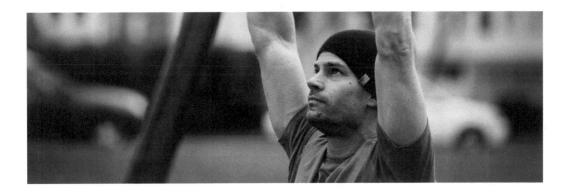

A WARM WELCOME

My name is Mike and I'm going to change your life. Actually, I'm going to help you change your life. Or perhaps I'm going to give you some things to think about that you may in turn act upon. In any case, I'm here to help. Over the years I've collected what I believe to be the most important and actionable mindset and habit components of meaningful transformation and boiled them down into 50 bite-sized concepts. A template to shift your thoughts, perceptions, and narratives when it comes to yourself, your food intake, your exercise and the habits that shape what you aspire to. It may be that what you read here gives you some new insights, re-enforces things you already know, challenges you, makes you slightly uncomfortable, gives you hope, a spark or a different way to look at things. You may nod your head, shake your head, be awestruck or "meh-struck." Whoever you are, whatever your situation or circumstance; however you have come across this publication—thank you. Thank you for being here. Thank you for reading. This book is for YOU. For the person who is frustrated by multiple attempts at weight loss and health improvements —this is for you. Welcome. For the person new to the idea of body transformation—this is for you. Welcome. For the seasoned enthusiast looking for new ideas, re-enforcement, re-affirmation and learning a few nuggets along the way—this is for you. Welcome. For the health and fitness coaches, nutrition professionals, physicians and other healthcare professionals looking to help clients and patients—this is for you. Welcome. In a nutshell, if you are looking for meaningful, sustainable fat loss and health enhancement or trying to help others on this journey, this book is for you. This isn't a typical "weight loss", "diet" or "body transformation" book. I'm here to ignite a flame of self-discovery; Discovering why you may have been unsuccessful in the past. Discovering how to look at the bigger picture of health, fat loss and transformation. Discovering your capabilities and potential. Discovering the power of mindset and habit transformation in changing your world. Discovering your path towards phenomenal health and a leaner frame.

ABOUT MIKE

With over 20 years of practical experience as a personal trainer, online weight loss coach and writer, Mike has continuously sought out the best ways to help people achieve sustainable success from a mindset and habits-first perspective. Along the way he has orchestrated effective, individualized solutions to thousands of clients both in person and around the world.

Mike has gained national and international attention for his philosophies on body composition, healthy habits, youth fitness and other topics relating to fitness and nutrition education. He has appeared on TV, print, numerous podcasts and has written over 400 online articles. Mike is the author of the well-received e-book *Talking Back to Diet Gurus: An Un-revolutionary and Un-Sexy Guide to Fat Loss*.

What a time to be alive. We are all here on this planet trying to navigate a perfect crap-storm of unfavorable evolutionary wiring in a modern environment of over-abundance. A contemporary world where technology has simultaneously negated much of our need to move while keeping us glued to alluring devices. Add to this disastrous double impact, a societal culture promoting idealized bodies and a diet culture promoting extreme quick fixes pumping out a steady stream of conflicting and contradictory half truths, mistruths and just plain lies.

We are up against it. No question. Westernized cultures face an obesity and ill-health epidemic to which there are no easy answers. The long-term success rates of weight loss are less than encouraging with 90%+ failing to keep weight off long term. And yet our society attempts to blame a singular dietary force (carbs, gluten, sugar, animal products, fat), shame us for our lack of willpower or pin it on our lack of knowledge, blame government, Big Food or other external forces. Our health world is one of glaring contradictions. At no point in history have we ever had more access to information on health, diet and fitness. Gyms, gym membership, healthy meal delivery services, tracking, fitness, nutrition and habit apps have all proliferated over the past decade and yet none of these factors have put a dent in our health or our waistlines.

As the noted author of *Grit: The Power of Passion and Perseverance*, Angela Duckworth puts it, "The one problem that really confronts humanity in the 21st century is humanity itself." Our collective and personal health is dictated by a complex and nuanced collection of factors related to our biology, genetics, epigenetics, psycho-socioeconomic and environmental elements. Our health can be transformed only through taking a wide lense, multifaceted and personal approach.

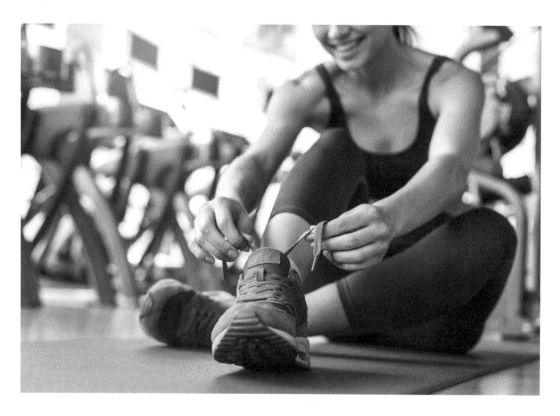

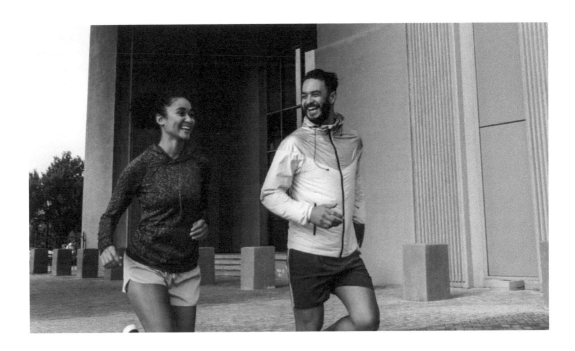

WHERE ARE WE GOING?

So much of the lean-minded approach is about taking a step back, taking a few deep breaths and deciding to cut through all the BS and forge your own path. This guide is a beacon—a navigational compass to help you carve out a healthy life. It's a manifesto of how to change your story. It's a nest of comfort in a journey that will be inherently uncomfortable. We are going to take a deeper dive into the bedrock of mindset, habit change and map out actionable precepts. Think of this guide as a transformation template; a completely personalizable infrastructure that you can refer to over and over again as needed.

Here's the straight goods: Sustainable fat loss isn't about eliminating categories of foods or eating particular ones. It's about rewiring your brain while developing solid, repeatable habits in a way that complements, not dominates your life. Essentially long term fat loss and better health comes down to aligning; heart, mind, and environment. The answer to fat loss and health will never be found in a bookstore, a documentary, or on Instagram —nor will it be delivered from a stage. It is a process. A journey. It is a constant dynamic and nuanced journey that will test you -

over and over again. Here's where fat loss and health CAN be found. It is found in self-forgiveness. It is found in abandoning the idea that there is a quick fix. It is found in developing an internal locus of control. It is found in the acceptance that your journey will take discipline, hard work, and patience. It is found in the realization that it is a journey to begin with (not a temporary goal with an end date). It is found in the firm belief that your health is sacred and part of your values systems. It is found in the acceptance that you will have setbacks. It is found in the belief that you are worth the time and effort (so are those close to you). It is found in making peace with your relationship with, and perceptions of food and exercise. I'm here to offer you a guide towards sifting through the BS (diet industry BS, and your own BS—you will encounter both).

Your ultimate success will be the culmination of the "4 P's"; Presence, Persistence, Patience, Practice.

All 4 of these components have to become part of the tapestry of your mindset and permeate into your actions—imperfect, but there.

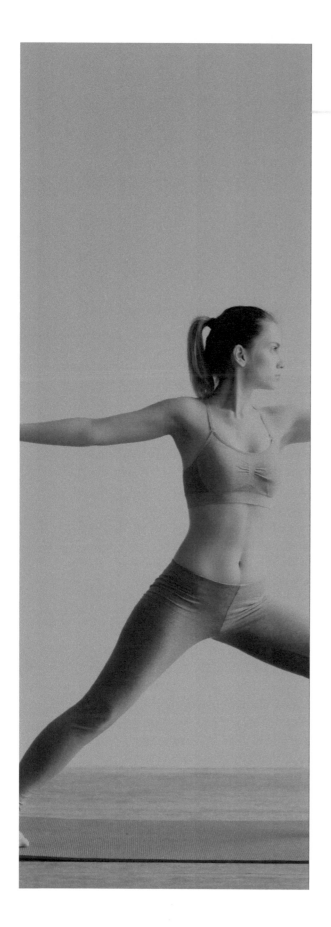

THE INSIDE-OUT APPROACH YOU NEED

This book contains very few nutritional prescriptives, no training regimens, no diets and no rules or constraints. In fact, my mandate is to REMOVE constraints and perceived barriers that you may be clinging to. I'm here to show you reasons why you can succeed—show you what is possible—show you how to think about your journey, rather than what to think. I want to take you on a path of self-discovery, self-acceptance, adaptation and self-identity. Instead of focusing on nutrition and exercise science, I'm going to draw from disciplines such as neurobiology, cognitive psychology, behavioral economics and weave it into the most vital thoughts, strategies and user-friendly tools to form a bulletproof foundation for success.

I'm here not as some cape-wearing guru with epic promises, nor will I tell you that everything you've heard about weight loss is wrong. I'm certainly not here to pitch you on some unique system of effortless transformation. Frankly, I have too much respect for you and your intelligence. I'm here to equip you, or perhaps help you see how well equipped you already are. I'm here to give you the metaphorical scalpel to perform the neuroplastic surgery necessary to kick some serious butt in losing fat, gaining health and improving your life. No hyperbole, no empty promises, no "hacks"—just a customizable blueprint for your own road towards success. So buckle up; read these one day at a time, in chunks or binge-read the whole thing at once. Ask questions, challenge your self-perceptions, challenge your perceived limitations and yes, challenge me on my perceptions of things. But most of all I want you to absorb, re-absorb and apply this to your own personal situation. Let it permeate and manifest into action.

PART 1: MINDSET
DAY 1: WELCOME TO YOUR NEW LIFE

Your new life. Let that sink in for a moment. Bask in the profundity of those words. Whether this is a brand new paradigm, a reset or anything in between—fully take in the impact of it all. This is a re-birth. You are embarking on a journey of health and self-improvement.

The time has come for you to show up for you. You've come to a fork in the road where you have made a definitive decision to take excellent care of your body (the only one you will ever have). This is the day you decide to (or re-commit to) making your health a priority. This is the day that you begin to realize your potential. This is the day you give your past failures, your resistance and self-doubt the middle finger. This is the day you turn a wish list item into a conscious and affirmative decisions. Today you embrace your potential, today you commit to weathering the storms.

Today you commit to editing your story. Excited? Good. Scared as hell? Also good. That's right, it's ok and even a GOOD thing that you are scared. Change (especially big change) IS scary.

Your feelings are perfectly valid. You don't want to fail again, you've had negative experiences when it comes to dieting and exercise, you live a busy and stressful life, you've been discouraged and life may have given you a few swift kicks to the nether-regions. It's ok to be scared. But today, And from now on, you will not succumb to that fear, you will cease to listen to the voices telling you to give up, telling you to start tomorrow, or Monday or January 1st.

Today is the first day of the rest of your life. Buckle up, the ride will be a bumpy one, but ultimately rewarding. You deserve the opportunity to strive for better health. Embrace the new you, embrace the discomfort, accept that it will be imperfect but know that you are fully capable.

Action Point: On a scale of 1-10, rate your confidence in being able to accomplish your desired level of fitness, weight loss or health goals? Have a number in mind.

Have a number in mind? Great. Why did you not choose the number below that one? Think about your answer and let it simmer.

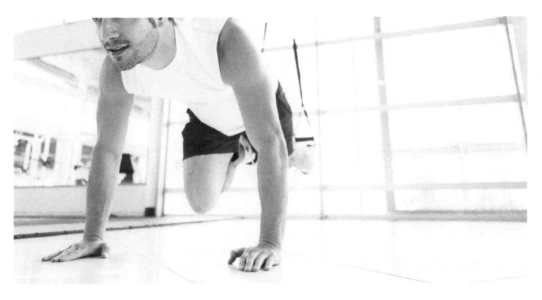

5

I've been largely inspired by the works of author Stephen Pressfield In his book *Do the Work*, he introduces two crucial concepts when it comes to fulfilling our life's purpose. The first is a metaphoric "invisible door"—an "attitude adjustment chamber" of sorts. In essence, when you take this health journey, there are elements that you have to leave behind if you are to succeed. Here is a partial list of things you have to leave at this metaphoric door;

Your excuses
Your bad attitude
Your fear
Your self-entitlement
Your hopes
Your anger

And hey, we all have some degree of one or more of the above. This isn't about having a perfect mindset or an unblemished slate going into this, nor is it about carrying zero negativity. After all we can't simply flip a switch to fix years of unhelpful conditioning. This is more about acknowledging that we may carry some of the above and that we need to work hard to squelch it. So here's what you DO get to take with you. In fact, here is what you MUST take with you as you traverse through this invisible door. These are the only 3 prerequisites you need for meaningful change.

Prerequisite 1: A passion for your health. At the risk of sounding hyperbolic, this is everything. This MUST be important to you— Like VERY important. If your health isn't ultimately important to you, this will be incredibly difficult to impossible to sustain. If you are reading this reluctantly (i.e. your spouse, your doctor, your friend recommended it) and it's simply an abstract idea or even a passing interest, I will advise you to step back and take a look at look at the big picture of life and where your health currently fits into that. I offer the following with compassion, empathy and non-judgement. Being "passionate" about your health has nothing to do with your current health or current state. It simply means you have an undeniable desire to be healthy.

Come as you are—we are all here to learn and better ourselves. You may be hesitant due to past experiences and don't want to fail. I understand. I've been there and so have many hundreds of thousands. This is the difference between interest and commitment (quote credit: Kenneth Blanchard). Interest is dipping a toe or a foot in the water, commitment is jumping in; fully immersing yourself, even when you aren't a strong swimmer. Even if the water is cold, murky, choppy or otherwise uncomfortable. Keep reading to equip yourself with the proverbial swimming lessons, water wings and wetsuit.

Prerequisite 2: A belief that you have control over the outcome. This is what psychology nerds call an "internal locus of control" or "agency"—a trust that you have a lot of say in what happens to you from a health-related standpoint. The opposite of this is an external locus of control—a belief that you are a passive recipient of your health and life destiny. Don't get me wrong here, we are all dealt a different hand in life. Some will have struggles beyond their control whether that be disease, disability or other genetic disadvantages. There are circumstances that may in fact make your life and ergo, your health pursuits more challenging. This doesn't mean you won't have self-doubt, moments of uncertainty or frustration. It does mean, however, that you are continually equipping yourself with the skills and mindset to know that you are in control. To quote my dear friend and mentor Brian Grasso:

"You may not know what you are capable of, just know you are fully capable."

Prerequisite 3: A resolve to never give up—no matter what. This will be an imperfect journey. Take that to the bank. What makes this kick at the can different is that this time you won't give up—no matter what. You will have breaks, setbacks, rebound weight gain, plateaus and a variety of frustrations. This time, however you will push past them, deal with them, take them in stride and you will NOT quit. The Navy Seals recruit training week is one of the most vigorous physical and mental challenges one could face; inhuman physical challenges, sleep deprivation, temperature extremes and other tests that push the limits of human capability. In the middle of the training ground of what's termed "beast barracks" is a bell. Recruits are told that at any time during the training they can bow out and ring the bell. I'm going to get you to start thinking about why you won't ring that bell. If at any time you feel like you want to give up,

I'll encourage you to ask these Four questions:

1. Would you be happy if you gave up and your life remained the same?
2. What's the worst that could happen if you keep going and don't achieve your goal?
3. How would it feel to tell other people (your children, your significant other, or good friends) why you gave up?
4. If you were to remain the same way you are now, would that genuinely make you happier? Let these questions marinade into your psyche.

Resistance: Time to Strike Back

You will face an invisible force along the way called resistance. The following is again a modification of Steven Pressfield's book Do the Work. Resistance has many faces including:

Fear	Distraction
Self-doubt	Timidity
Procrastination	Ego
Addiction	

Resistance is invisible. It cannot be seen, heard, touched, or smelled but it can be felt. Resistance is a repelling force. Resistance aims to kill. Its target is the epicenter of our being—in this case our desire for better health. We are in a fight to the death. Do whatever you can... whatever you MUST to resist resistance.

This is where our narratives are so important. As soon as any doubt, insecurity, de-motivation, complacency, or distraction hits—fight back. Bite resistance in the ass. If you wait for inspiration to strike, you will lose... you need to strike inspiration first and often.

> Action Point: Can you answer a definitive "yes" to the three prerequisites you need to have to make meaningful change:
> 1. Do you have a passion for your health?
> 2. Do you believe that you have control over the outcome?
> 3. Are you prepared to never give up—no matter what?

Here's the thing; you are designed to be healthy. Your body is a vessel meant to move and to eat nutrient-dense foods. Somewhere along the line our society, our thrifty genes, our environment, our thoughts and our circumstances have conspired to lead us astray. When you begin to shape habits and feel better, you are not only making a myriad of positive physical and mental health shifts, but you are also becoming closer to who you are MEANT to be. You are designed to shape your life in a way that is fulfilling and healthy.

With that in mind, you are also fully deserving of the pursuit of better health. I encourage being appropriately selfish when it comes to this pursuit—this is essential to achieving better health and leaning out. I work with a lot of mothers, single parents, people with aging relatives and those with dependents on both ends of the age spectrum (the so-termed "sandwich generation"). I often hear how little time and energy people have and that they barely have the physical and emotional resources to take care of others—let alone themselves.

Regardless of your situation, your busy life or your responsibility for dependents, carving time out for you is paramount. You will be of much better service to those around you when you take care of yourself. Find the time, MAKE the time, ask for help from others and do everything in your power to put yourself in a position to be more healthy.

Convey to your children, your friends, your boss and your significant other that you need some time for self-care—of which exercise and healthy eating is central. Be brave and communicate your needs, don't be afraid to say "no" and don't be afraid to schedule workouts and see them as "sacred" appointments.

Action point: I'm going to challenge you to think about when you can schedule time for yourself and how you are going to let others know that you need to prioritize yourself. I'm going to ask you especially to muster up the conviction and boldness to declare to yourself and others that you are 100% worthy of time to work on your health.

You are not your scale weight/dress size/health status. Repeat this message to yourself as often as needed. It may be that this message will take a longer time to sit well with you. Our society has placed so much value on outward appearance—lionizing smaller, and otherwise shredded athletic bodies. There is pressure from all angles to look a certain way and when we don't fit into this social box of hotness, it's often looked upon as a character defect—a weakness of will, a sign of laziness or apathy.

Self-love and self-acceptance must be at the forefront of your journey. You may be in a place where you have been beaten yourself up over your indulgences, your weight or your fitness level. I am going to ask you in a very serious way to shift your narrative towards self-acceptance. When that self-flagellating mindset begins to rear its ugly head, counter it.

"I am already amazing. I may struggle with my weight or healthy habits right now, but I'm working hard on my health. I will screw this up from time to time and when I do, I will forgive myself AND get right back into my healthy lifestyle."

Please note that his does not mean that you are accepting your situation. In fact you should be dissatisfied with your situation—but only because you deserve better for yourself. Part of loving yourself is accountability. It's okay to want better for yourself, it's also okay to have aesthetic goals—there is nothing wrong with wanting to look better naked. As long as these are YOUR goals and not a reflection of society's version of perfection. Acceptance is not resignation—it's not accepting defeat. Acceptance is meeting reality where it is and then fully experiencing it. Fully feel your emotions around your situation, while focusing on what you can do right now.

Here is a handy chart to help sort out what self-forgiveness is and what it is not.

SELF-FORGIVENESS IS	SELF-FORGIVENESS IS NOT
Taking your goals seriously while shunning the need for perfection	Not taking your goals seriously
Feeling disappointed in yourself but not beating yourself up over missteps.	Going easy on yourself
Doing the best you can for yourself knowing you won't win every battle.	Giving yourself an "out" each time temptation strikes under the guise of "forgiveness."
Choosing self-love even if it's counterintuitive right now.	An absence of knee jerk feelings of guilt. These emotions will happen.

Self-forgiveness is about setting yourself up for long-term success mentally and emotionally by being kind to yourself. You can simultaneously practice self-acceptance and self-improvement. This means accepting strengths, weaknesses, talents and flaws.

Action point: When you experience moments of beating yourself up, I'm going to ask you to take a moment to remind yourself that self-compassion comes first. Practice taking things in stride, learning from slips and responding with determination and action instead of a cycle of self-loathing.

I'm also going to have you list 3 things you are great at. This could be a hobby, skill or another attribute. Bask in this for a few moments. You have a lot to offer this world.

Honest self-reflection is the "yang" to the self-acceptance "yin." Self-compassion is central and so is self-reflection. It's time to take honest stock of your situation—full length mirror check time. Meaningful change can only take place once you've admitted to yourself that you aren't doing all you can to keep yourself healthy. Be honest with yourself, but also be gentle and forgiving. Here are some questions you can mull over.

Evaluate, re-evaluate, assess:

Am I acting in the healthiest way I can for myself?

Am I doing the best I can for my body?

Am I REALLY eating healthfully or do I just think I am?

Am I lifting weights a few times per week?

Am I getting intentional movement daily?

Am I being honest about my indulging?

Am I passing off bad habits as "everything in moderation"?

And then..

What can I do now to take better care of myself?

The digging and scrutiny might give you a temporary case of the "blah's." On a personal level, just writing these words actually prompted some fleeting negative emotions; guilt, inadequacy, self-loathing. This isn't necessarily a bad thing—provided we take those emotions as our body and brain's signal to take action. Now go and re-read day 3; practice self-compassion, self-forgiveness and self-love as you embark on (or re-commit to) your health journey. This isn't about dwelling on your current situation or past failures—it's about taking stock of your current reality and processing how you can make some improvements. Starting now.

Action point: What is one behavior you feel is sabotaging your health? What's one thing you can change right now that will further your health?

DAY 6: WE ARE IRRATIONAL
(AND THAT MAKES US HUMAN)

We need to attack change at the deepest level. One of the most formidable obstacles to change is that we are not inherently logical beings. Of the many ways we delude ourselves, perhaps our biggest self-deception is that we think logically. The hard truth we need to accept is that our day-to-day decisions are largely the result of emotion, not logic. We gather information not to make a decision, but to justify a decision we have already made. We are products of ancient brains in a society of abundance and convenience.

Part of the journey is stepping back and looking at the big picture aspects of our brain and how it operates. It's realizing that most of what we think is a perception—not the objective reality of things. Perhaps the biggest impairment to self-improvement is that we don't know what we don't know. To quote David McRaney, author of *You are Not so Smart: etc,* "We are unreliable narrators in the story of our lives."

I'll focus on one of the more glaring cognitive blind spots we succumb to, what behavioral economists call the "current moment bias" or "temporal discounting." This means that we gravitate towards a "take what's available now," scarcity-oriented default. Furthermore, we pretty much suck at both predicting a future scenario and how we will respond to said scenario. We are a society of instant gratification—prone to the roller coaster swings of hedonic adaptation. We seek immediate reward in the current moment, while leaving the uncomfortable stuff for later—even if we know cognitively the long-term reward is greater.

A 1998 study confirmed the old adage, "The road to hell is paved with good intentions." When asked what they would choose a week from that point when they became hungry, 74% of participants said they'd choose fruit over junk food but when the day arrived, 70% chose chocolate.

Your journey of health and leaning out will be one of gaining self-awareness. Awareness of your thoughts and how you act on them, awareness of your vulnerabilities, strengths, triggers and how you respond in given situations.

> **Action point:** I'm going to encourage you to practice taking a step back and to pay attention to thoughts, feelings, and actions surrounding food, training, lifestyle and personal relationships. I'm going to challenge you to delay gratification, to throw a proverbial wrench in the brain's stimulus/response cycle. I'm going to get you to say "wait a minute, let me pay attention to what's going on here." I'm going to have you reflect on situations and ask "does this benefit my journey right now?" Practice this for the next 24 hours from this moment.

Instead of inspiring yourself into the right action, act your way into the right inspiration. We tend to get things backwards when looking at the sequence of events that lead to successful outcomes. We've bought into this illusion that we must be "inspired" or "motivated" to act on something. This is unmitigated BS. If we only act when we "feel" motivated, nothing substantial will ever be accomplished.

What is your biggest source of resistance? Fear? Self-doubt? Timidity? Ego? Addiction? Where does this come from? Fight the distractions, battle your personal resistance— strike first, strike often. Action often precedes inspiration. Whatever you do, do not be paralyzed into inaction. MOVE, buy some produce and eat it. The best way to combat resistance is to take immediate action.

Not just any action, however—committed and valued action. Valued actions are those actions that align with your values. And because you are reading this, I will assume that health is a strong value for you.

Is it hard to act when you don't feel like it? Yep. So while my coaching style is more nurturing than drill sergeant, this is one of a handful of instances where there is no coddling/shortcuts. You have to put your big boy/big girl pants on and just act. You aren't alone in procrastinating on this first step, but this is what will get you closer to your goal.

Momentum trumps motivation—always. Start before you are ready. Don't think—act! Showing up is 90% of the battle. Showing up to exercise, showing up to prepare healthy meals, showing up when it comes to self-reflection.

By getting moving you will feel more like moving. Don't wait until you feel like moving. Don't wait until you are inspired to grocery shop, don't wait for the right motivational quote to hit the gym, stop waiting for the Dalai Lama to tell you to relax and be grateful. Take that first step and take it now—however small that step may be.

Choose "day one" over "one day."
Mel Robbins, a prominent speaker and author wrote a fantastic book called *The 5 Second Rule*. Her theory is that once you have an inkling to do something, act on it— right away. The backbone of the theory being you will have about 5 seconds before your brain tries to trick you out of it and divert you to a less productive action instead. The key thing initially (and perpetually) is to develop the triggers and disruptions to lead towards action. As soon as your ancient, impulsive brain says, "Hey, maybe not now," shut it down, take a productive action—however small. Tell whatever source of resistance that is holding you back to EFF off—not this time. This is a big part of the rewiring, re-directing process.

Robbins claims we need a jolt of what she calls "activation energy"—a scientific principle by which the amount of energy required to initiate a chemical reaction that is greater than the amount of energy needed to sustain it.

Continuously Seek out the M.E.A (Minimal Enjoyable Action)

If you are really struggling to get things right, it may be time to find your MEA. Those 5k runs too much? DO them as a walk/run. Or just walk. Meal prepping 21 meals a week insurmountable? Prep 3 days out of 7, or just dinners. MEA is about scaling back when necessary. It's about starting power, one thing, one small step. MEA provides you with the reinforcement of a habit while giving you a hit of dopamine—igniting the reward centers in your brain for your accomplishment.

The real meat of this is: don't wait for inspiration to strike. You will have to strike at inspiration first and you will have to strike hard and strike often. You will have to commit to an offensive approach when it comes to getting healthy food in your mouth, getting intentional activity and overall doing things to make you feel more fulfilled.

Action point: Now get out there and do something that furthers your health—before you do anything else. Step away from day 8, step away from your phone, laptop or TV remote. Walk, cut up a pepper, eat some cherry tomatoes, do some squats.

DAY 8: KICK YOURSELF IN THE COMFORT ZONE (WITHOUT BEATING THE CRAP OUT OF IT)

Any undertaking requires change. In many cases, such change will be uncomfortable. You are going to have to work for this. sweat for this.. compromise and sacrifice for this. You will not, however, have to be in pain, in constant deprivation or misery. This should complement, not take over your life.

The more we desire a certain food/behavior, the more deeply we have to think about how it will impact our health.

This will mean different things to different people but here are some examples of how you might give your comfort zone a jab:

- Go to bed 30 minutes earlier
- Grocery shop religiously on a specific day
- Bring 1 healthy meal or snack with you when you leave your home
- Walk 2000 steps more per day
- Go to the gym 3 times per week (even if you don't stay long or work out hard)
- Drink a bottle of water at work or home
- Say no to the tasty food you normally always say yes to (or say yes without guilt, but say no more often)
- Drive right past the drive thru

The above may not seem revolutionary, but rest assured when practiced consistently it is surprisingly effective. A kick in the comfort zone.

Our diet and quick fix culture would have you believe you must eliminate entire categories of foods to lose weight and heal all ailments. This would be kicking the crap out of your comfort zone—and not conducive to long-term success.

So while I won't delve too deeply into the "what to eat" territory, I will say that sustainable changes are best accomplished through flexible dieting. My dietary approach to fat loss is essentially picking the best eating pattern that gets you into a calorie deficit in the least soul-sucking way possible. While some can thrive on more rigid eating patterns, being too stringent can backfire for most. If you have a lot of weight to lose, losing weight rapidly through a more strict eating pattern can be effective, however it has to be a way of eating you can sustain.

The vast majority of people, however CAN in fact make excellent, sustainable progress through:

- Switching to mostly whole, minimally processed foods—including lots of vegetables
- Eating moderately high protein
- Getting adequate sleep
- Eating more satiating carbs as well as beans and legumes
- Eating out less
- Drinking more water
- Intentional movement
- Strength training
- Indulgences here and there

Fasting !

Simple, but not necessarily easy. Much easier, however than eliminating entire categories of foods and having to adhere to strict and otherwise arbitrary rules that today's diets are so fond of.

The good news is that just about everything you are going to read in this book is designed specifically to set you up to consistently follow through on the above.

Action Point: What is one way you feel you need to get uncomfortable? Do this thing today.

DAY 9: YOUR TRANSFORMATION: THE NEGOTIABLE VS THE NON-NEGOTIABLE

One of the hallmarks of long term success is that we have some say over how things are accomplished. As mentioned, diet culture proposes all-or-nothing approaches with rigid guidelines and immutable rules to abide by (all the while telling you, the consumer, that their diet is "easy" to follow. LOL).

One of the truths about your personal journey of health is that it will require the aforementioned "kick in the comfort zone." The how and when and other such details, however, are largely negotiable. Here are some examples:

FAT LOSS NON-NEGOTIABLE VS NEGOTIABLE

NON-NEGOTIABLE	NEGOTIABLE
✔ Disrupting your comfort zone	✔ HOW you disrupt your comfort zone
✔ Intentional movement	✔ Your form of exercise
✔ Eating in a calorie deficit	✔ The method/diet you use to get into a deficit
✔ Eating vegetables	✔ The kind of veggies you eat
✔ Drinking water	✔ Other non-caloric liquids you consume
✔ Strength training	✔ Sets/reps scheme/program
✔ Creating awareness of intake	✔ Counting calories
✔ Self-forgiveness	✔ Your own style of constructive self-reflection
✔ Restraint when it comes to indulging	✔ The type of indulgences you choose

Action Point: I will expand on many of these points on future days. For now, I'll encourage you to think about how you want to disrupt your comfort zone. Focus on realistic, challenging tasks and begin to take action on those tasks. Think about how you can set your life up in a way that it is easier to accomplish these processes.

DAY 10: THIS IS GOING TO SUCK (AT TIMES) AND YOU ARE GOING TO SUCK AT IT (AT FIRST)

Real talk time. A hands-on-your-shoulders, look you in the eye and lovingly and gently deliver some tough-to-swallow pills kind of talk.

We've been enticed into believing that body transformation is effortless, fast and permanent. This is the "unholy trinity" of diet industry promises. Here are some hard truths about the journey, followed by some not-so-gloomy messages of hope. In my many years as a fitness and weight management coach, I've seen countless people quit their journey early because they hit a stumbling block, became frustrated by their lack of follow-through or some other line of reasoning that was well within their control.

Fundamentally, fat loss and significant improvements in health require more change than we might expect. While it doesn't necessarily require huge, overnight change, the consistency it requires within the context of small changes is almost always underestimated.

- It requires making a healthier decision FAR more often than not.
- It requires making a choice to create a healthy meal and do a workout when you are tired, stressed (or both) FAR more often than not.
- It requires saying "no" more often than you will be comfortable with.
- It requires defaulting to physical activity more times than not.
- It requires quitting something that is detracting from your progress. This could be a nightly Netflix binge, mindless scrolling, video gaming, etc. (You don't have to swear off any of the aforementioned, but you may have to cut back).
- It requires hanging out less with people who pull you off track.
- It requires framing your goals through the lens of sacrifice, not wish lists.It requires the realization that while each situation is unique, your particular problems are not.
- It requires examining and challenging your current belief systems about yourself, your capabilities and the mindset that might be holding you back.
- It requires accepting that your shortage of movement and absence of progress is due to lack of priority, not lack of time.
- It requires prioritizing sleep; finding ways to get more and better quality rest.
- It requires some form of tracking; whether you track food intake, weight, girth, etc.
- It requires you to NOT give scale fluctuations any emotional value. You will need to mostly detach from the minor up and down fluctuations you will see from day to day or week to week.

You will get frustrated, you will want to quit, you will temporarily fail...likely several times.

Please focus on the word "temporarily" here.

But There's Good News in all of this. And this is more powerful than any of the aforementioned reality checks.

- The benefits of your hard work and consistency will pay off in more ways than you can possibly imagine. (Read this a few times, please.)
- Things do get easier and more ingrained the more you do them.
- While you can't change the fact that things will be uncomfortable, you can reframe the discomfort as something to embrace—or at least continuously accept.
- When you do fail, you have the capability to be forgiving of yourself.. And keep going —no matter what.
- Being 100% committed to your health doesn't mean you will be 100% compliant.
- While losing fat and improving health won't necessarily make you happier, it WILL make you stronger, more confident and better equipped to face life as you age.
- Even when you don't see the manifestation of your results on the scale or tape, you ARE making changes at the molecular level to your health.
- You are becoming an amazing role model for those around you (your children, your loved ones, your friends, your co-workers).
- You now identify as a person who takes their health seriously. Eating well and moving often are now just aligning to your personal values system.

Remember that your journey will take consistent practice. Any new endeavor does. Do not expect to be immediately amazing at food prep, strength training, time-management, sleep management. I wouldn't hand you a harpsichord and expect you to be able to knock out a perfect "Minuet in G Major." What I'm saying is expect to struggle, expect to fail but insist on your own persistence.

Embrace the failures; learn and grow from them. The pathway we have trouble seeing is often the most productive and progressive one. Work hard on reframing your missteps as growth opportunities.

Action Point: Think about the next time you have to make a decision that will impact your health; make a conscious decision to go against what you would normally do, what you have done in the past. Make the decision that will further your health. For example: Normally slink into a comfortable couch and grab a bag of Doritos? Go for a walk instead.

One of the most striking factors when it comes to sustained success in any venture is a concept known as "grit." Grittiness is essentially having perseverance and passion for long-term goals. It's being able to stick with something despite it being difficult or otherwise mundane.

Angela Duckworth—a leader in the field of grit has uncovered (through years of research) that the smartest, the most talented or most athletic are not necessarily the highest achievers. It's those with perseverance, resilience and the resolve to improve that do.

So are you frustrated? GOOD.
Duckworth has this to say about it:

"Frustration is probably a sign that you're on the right track and need to gut it out through the natural human aversion to mental effort and feeling overwhelmed so you can evolve."

Allow yourself to feel frustrated but instead of dwelling on it, show up differently, resolve to conquer and keep conquering.

Doing repeated scales was boring to me when I took piano lessons. Repeated vanilla-looking front kicks and left jabs were definitely not the 360 Van Damme-esque spin kicks I wanted to learn. Later in life I would learn the importance of what researcher Daniel Chambliss calls "the mundanity of excellence." Chambliss conducted a landmark study on the success of swimmers. His basic premise suggests that "excellence" is overrated. He describes excellence in a way that seems mundane—rejecting the idea that an athlete possess "natural talent." He instead suggests that an athlete achieves excellence due to a variety of other factors that are often mistaken and mislabeled as God-given talent.

Chambliss theorizes:
"The actions themselves are not special; the care and consistency with which it is made is."

His basic premise being that Olympic swimmers and club team recreational swimmers are far more alike than not.

Malcolm Gladwell's *Outliers* emphasizes the importance of time honing your craft, proposing an oft-cited (and oft-contested) Ten Thousand Hour Rule (that it takes a minimum of ten thousand hours to become an expert at any given subject matter).

Success comes down to nailing the basics. The boring, repetitive and uninteresting basics.

One way to improve on the fundamentals is to reduce variety—an idea that at first might seem counterintuitive.

Anecdotally, my clients who require a great deal of variety and excitement in meals and exercise selection have the hardest time out of the gate achieving results. I'm not suggesting food has to be bland and you have to relegate yourself to only the stationary bike and planks. What I am saying is be open to embracing less variety. Be open to the idea that reducing your choices can actually help you better establish habits. Be open to the idea that mastering the basics of cooking and exercise technique will open the doors to more proficiency when branching out.

By all means seek out new recipes, add some spices and try out exercise variations. But put your mental energies into the consistency of healthy eating and movement first and foremost—knowing that yep, you'll be eating things that don't taste like chocolate chip cookies most of the time. You'll learn to embrace the mundanity as you see the effect it has on your life.

Action Point: Remind yourself of your purpose, your health-related interests and that anything deeply important to you is going to have to be fought for. Remind yourself that this is a long and bumpy road and the only way to achieve what you want is to stick to your lifestyle consistently over the long run. Take that extra walk, do that extra day in the gym, prepare that extra salad, actively play with your children those extra minutes.

According to Duckworth, one of the best ways to develop and foster grit is to develop a growth mindset. Carol Dwek's book *Mindset: The New Psychology of Success* is a groundbreaking book about how different mindsets can elicit vastly different outcomes. This concept has become popular in childhood education efforts and is making some noise in the self-help world as well. Here is a rundown of growth vs fixed mindsets:

- A "fixed mindset" assumes that our character, intelligence, and creative ability are static givens which we can't change in any meaningful way.
- A "growth mindset," on the other hand, thrives on challenge and sees failure not as evidence of unintelligence but as a heartening springboard for growth and for stretching our existing abilities.

Out of these two mindsets, which we manifest from a very early age, springs a great deal of our behavior, our relationship with success and failure in both professional and personal contexts, and ultimately our capacity for happiness.

In your health pursuits it is vital to nurture a growth mindset. This will keep you resilient and gritty—equipping you for long-term success. It's easy to catch yourself slipping into a fixed mindset in the early going or when the going gets tough. Here are some reframes to some deceptive brain messages you may encounter:

FIXED MINDSET	GROWTH MINDSET
Ugh I can never resist the sweets—I have no self-control.	Well I ate more sweets than I had planned, but I'll find a better way to cope with my stress next time
I'm so winded every time I try and run —I'm not cut out for this.	I know I'll get better through walk/run programs. It's slow progress but it's progress.
I just can't get myself out of bed in time to make food for the day.	What I'm currently doing isn't working but I'm going to find a way to make it work.
I get super hungry at night and I overeat. It's a cycle I just can't break.	I notice I'm really hungry at night. I'm going to find a way around that.
I'm so uncoordinated, I feel silly doing strength training.	It feels awkward right now but that's because I'm new at it. I'll keep practicing.

Seeing yourself as someone capable of change, progress and knowing you have a lot of say in how healthy you can become is a crucial step to sustained success.

Action point: What is something you feel you simply cannot do when it comes to improving your health? Challenge this assumption and flip it on its head. Declare and proclaim that you underestimated your own abilities and reframe this from a growth mindset perspective.

"Comparison is the thief of joy"—Winston Churchill.

We live in a world of pervasive social media consumption. While the internet has open sourced information and communication, it has also open-sourced insecurity and a comparative mindset. Flipping through instagram feeds can be a disheartening experience. We are constantly exposing ourselves to other peoples' highlight reels—a virtual carousel of curated perfection. If you follow fitness people you will likely be inundated with lean, tanned, defined and scantily clad bodies, too-good-to-be true transformations, weight loss stories and superhuman athletic feats.

All of this can lead to feelings of not being good enough as well as setting unrealistic expectations and overly-lofty goals. It's not to say you shouldn't aim high and be ambitious with your objectives, but setting goals based on the standards of outliers is a recipe for discouragement and quitting early. Studies back this up—showing higher weight loss expectation as an independent factor in dropping out of a weight loss program.

I'm going to ask you to personalize and define (or redefine) what success means to you. Feel free to be ambitious, but make it personal to your situation, your life, your availability and time limitations. Feel free to aspire to a certain weight, dress size or a physical state you used to be in as an adult. I am going to ask you, however NOT to strive to look like someone else. Your body is your body. That woman on the cover of Cosmo or Woman's Health has a unique genetic predisposition and likely has a personal trainer, personal chef and all kinds of other support (not to mention perfect lighting, angles and airbrush treatments). Ultimately my wish is for you to aim for a healthier version of you—whatever that looks like.

We will discuss goal-setting mastery as an entire separate entity but I will encourage to include in your definition of success a strong leaning towards health-centric goals and what is known as "non-scale victories" (NSV's for short). Here is a list of NSV's you might consider striving for—in addition to your body composition goals.

- More energy
- Fewer cravings
- Less guilt when indulgences occur
- Increased weight you can push, pull, squat or move
- Improved libido
- Less pain

- Reduced/eliminated need for a medication
- Running a distance
- Completing a race
- Increased confidence
- Performing daily tasks with less effort

Weight loss as a goal is awesome—but realize the scale weight won't always go your way. There will be times where you need to look at all the other benefits your new lifestyle is reaping.

Action point: Write down your definition of success. Be sure to include at least 5 non-scale victories that you are shooting for.

Your self-talk is central to a healthy mindset. So much of who we are, whether or not we persevere is our inner voice—our personal narratives—how we frame and interpret events that happen to us. Your self-talk may be one of the most powerful tools in your arsenal of fat loss and improved health.

It's very possible that you have created some false narratives about yourself, your situation, your abilities or your potential. Experts estimate that we have anywhere from 12-60 THOUSAND thoughts per DAY. Of those thousands of thoughts, an estimated 80% of those are negative thoughts. And perhaps most striking—95% of our thoughts are on repeat. In short, we have a lot of negativity to fight against.

Re-framing from both a self-perception and situational standpoint is a monumental cog in the complex wheel of personal achievement. Your personal narrative and framing skills will help get you through the inevitable bumps in the road, it will strengthen your action-orientation, bolster your perseverance and will take you through the sticky points in life.

When I first started in the industry 20+ years ago I remember reading a quote that has stuck with me ever since. "Life is 10% what happens to us and 90% how we react to what happens to us." This Charles Swindoll quote resonated beyond words and began my own mindset transformation (a painstakingly slow, non-linear and drawn out, still-in-progress journey).

It's not you—it's your brain. It's a bizarre concept no doubt. But once we are able to wrap our heads around the fact that our minds and brains are separate entities we can help ourselves think logically in the face of temptation.

Dr. Jeffery Shwartz in his book, *You Are Not Your Brain* suggests a 4-step process in averting temptation. I will shorten this to 3 steps.

1. Identify the deceptive message: recognize the counterproductive thoughts, urges, desires and impulses.

2. Reframe the message: Change your perception of the importance of the brain messages—declare them deceptive. Remind yourself it's not you, it's your brain. They are emotional sensations, not true emotions.

3. Re-focus the message: Distract, detract and seek out your other options. Put your mental capacity into finding something else to occupy your hands and brain.

Your pain is real. Your struggle is real. The frustration is real. But the story that is causing it is something we make up and something we can change. The path of change is every bit as real and even more powerful than the struggle and frustration.

Action point: When those messages hit—the ones telling you to give in, telling you food will make you feel better right now, the ones telling you can't do something— approach them with a counter trigger. Declare them deceptive and turn the message around—get to the reality of the situation. The reality that you have power over your thoughts and emotions.

DAY 15: MANAGING YOUR SELF-TALK PART 2: REFRAMING WITH AGENCY

There is a surprising amount of power in using "I don't" vs "I can't." This small, yet profound switch can make all the difference in the world when it comes to consistently making great decisions about your health.

It comes down to the concept of locus of control. When you have an EXTERNAL locus of control, you believe that your life is mostly controlled by outside forces and factors and ergo you believe there is no point in putting forth effort in any meaningful venture. An INTERNAL locus of control, conversely is one where you feel like you have a great deal of sway when it comes to what happens to you. When you believe this, you are better equipped to take charge and be responsible for your actions and inactions.

To say "I can't" is to be a slave to some arbitrary rule whereas to declare "I don't" takes root who you are as a person—how you see yourself and your priorities. Other verbiage you might consider; "I choose to" or "I choose not to," "I am" or "I am not." The difference can be quite remarkable when it comes to quelling overeating. This study shows the power of agency as when students offered chocolate, those who said "I can't eat it" chose to eat the bar 61% of the time, as opposed to 36% from those who said "I don't eat it."

Here is a handy "cheat sheet" on how to reframe some common scenarios:

RE-FRAMING CHEAT SHEET

UNPRODUCTIVE	PRODUCTIVE
✖ I can't eat that	✔ I CHOOSE not to eat that
✖ I shouldn't eat that	✔ I CHOOSE to eat that and savor it
✖ I should wake up early to work out	✔ I will wake up early to workout
✖ I had 4 cookies...I have no self-control	✔ I had 4 cookies...it happened, it's okay-time to move forward
✖ I need to have one of those fresh donuts	✔ Not in the plan right now-some other time
✖ I won't have an hour to do my workout, I'll go tomorrow	✔ I CAN do a quick 30 minute workout
✖ Ah what the heck, its already been a bad week of eating, what's another day	✔ This week has been less than optimal, but i can turn it around starting now
✖ It's too early-I need to sleep	✔ I'm going to get up right now. I need the training more than I need sleep. I'll go to bed early tonight.

> **Action point:** Use the words "I choose not to" or "I don't" when you are faced with tempting items. Practice this form of taking control. Remember that you are the one who makes the calls. You have choices—commit to them.

DAY 16: MANAGING YOUR SELF-TALK PART 3: INTERROGATIVE SELF-TALK

I first read about this strategy while reading Daniel Pink's excellent book *Drive*. This is whereby instead of making a declarative statement such as "I can do this," one instead asks the question, "Can I do this?" So termed the "Bob the Builder" method (after the children's animated character whose catchphrase is "Can he build it?"), this strategy is more of a self-challenge. By asking the question, it activates the circuitry of the brain involved in thinking about the "how's" of the journey. When we think about the process, we map out specific action steps. It's the difference between an active and a passive cognitive response. Asking a question prompts action, whereas a declaration or a mantra prompts a passive response.

As an example; When you wake up in the morning, you may be thinking about how you will make healthy choices that day. By saying "I can do this," you are only temporarily revving yourself up—with no direction on specifics. By asking, "Can I do this?" you begin to think about ways in which you will execute. You may start to think about your opportunities—packing some healthy snacks, hitting a grocery store, ordering the chicken salad instead of the burger and fries.

So next time you are tempted to say, "I got this," ask a question instead.. And then map out the steps. Research has demonstrated much better follow-through on tasks with interrogative self-talk than declarative.

Action point: Whether faced with the decision to get to the gym or go for a run or to start cooking a healthy meal, ask yourself, "Can I do this"? Then come up with the resources as to why you can.

DAY 17: YOUR LANGUAGE ON HOW YOU INTERPRET EVENTS

In my 20+ years of counseling on weight loss, I can predict with about 95% accuracy whether someone will see results based on how they describe their week of eating. Pay attention to how your day/week has been going. Recall the honest self-reflection (Day 5) and kick in the comfort zone (day x) lessons.

Here are some examples of the type of dialogue you would want to hear from yourself if asked how your week went health-wise.

"It's been a great week."
"I did really well this week."
"It's been a good week." ("good" said with confidence).
"With rare exception, it was a healthy week of eating."

Here are some examples of the type of dialogue that will keep you stuck in place;

"The week was okay."
"Not a bad week."
"It was good." ("good" said cautiously or as a question)
"It's been an okay week."
"Had some good parts to it."

This is an observation, not a judgement. The reality is, however, that you will need to have more weeks like the above than below to consistently see results. Celebrate the fact that it may have been a "better than usual" week or day, but also be cognizant of the fact that "hit and miss" won't get you to where you want to be. Think about what will take your week from "not bad" to "great." Execute those things bit by bit.

It probably wouldn't hurt either to remind you of being "all in" versus testing the waters. The following scenario happens quite often; I will set out some specific guidelines for a client to follow. The client will respond with, "Okay, I'll give this a try." Stop right there. Rewind and reframe. "Yes, I will do this.", "Yes, I can do this."

I recognize it because I did this incessantly when tasked with something I found to be difficult. "I'll try" is tentative. It's non-committal, it smacks of hesitation. Remember the wisdom of Yoda here, "Do or do not, there is no try."

Action Point: Think about what types of habits and actions will get you to the dialogue of "great." Throughout the week, ask yourself if you are doing "okay" or "great." If it's "great"—keep that up. If it's "okay", what can you do to get that to "great"?

DAY 18: EXCUSE-PROOFING PART 1: "I HAVE ALL THE TIME IN THE WORLD"

This is the first of a 4-part series on "excuse-proofing." Our journey can be taken off track by our own justifications, perceived obstacles and flat-out excuses.

My job as your coach is not so much to call BS on you but rather to empower you to call BS on yourself. Believe me, I've used ALL of these excuses many times so I know how to spot them in myself now.

One of the most prominent self-deceptions we use as humans is the "it can wait" syndrome—which leads, of course to the notorious and oft-repeated, "I'll start tomorrow" rationale. This stems from two misconceptions about time:

1.We have copious amounts of it. Remember the part about humans being irrational? Well there is no better example of this than our perception of time and how much of it we have. We somehow delude ourselves into thinking there's always tomorrow. We put off reading Tolstoy, learning Spanish, taking piano lessons and yes, our health pursuits because we feel it can wait.

2. We will achieve our goals in the time we think it should take: This is what's called the "planning fallacy" popularized by legendary behavioral economist Daniel Kahneman. This misconception stems from an inherent mental flaw in our abilities to predict how long things will take and is bolstered by the diet culture's unrealistic and unsustainable "get thin quick" schemes. We have been conditioned to believe that weight loss should be fast—to the tune of 3-7 lbs a WEEK in some cases. This unfortunately leaves many people disappointed in what may otherwise should be considered significant results. There is no escaping the fact that transformation takes time, isn't linear and it will take longer than we think it might.

The time factor can also be related to what behavioral economists call "current moment bias" or "hyperbolic discounting." This is our human nature to take the instant reward now rather than putting in the effort and reaping the larger rewards later. Yummy cheesecake when we're trying to lose fat? Start the diet tomorrow. Get to the gym? Not when Netflix beckons.

This is a prime source of procrastination because we think we can always put something off to tomorrow. But what if it couldn't wait? What if we treated our health a little more urgently—not in a fear-based way but in a way that sparks action. What if the next time your mind defaults to "I'm too tired to workout" or "I'm too hungry/stressed to stop for groceries" we put our cognitive foot down and say, "Not today.".. Today, I will resist this urge. Today I will exert control over my health. Today I will do something to further my health instead of detract from it."

Making these decisions more often than not will lead to results—I guarantee it.

In a broader, reflect-on-life kind of way, I invite you to look at 2 ancient Greek concepts of time: chronos and kairos.

Chronos is essentially "chronological" time. A flowing river that passively carries us away. Kairos by contrast is a still lake which we swim in. In essence, chronos = quantity, kairos = quality. In any given moment we will experience time in both frames. In a big picture sense, seek the kairos in your life. Seek the kairos in your health pursuits—even the challenging ones. View your time as valuable, and opportunities to improve yourself as valuable.

There won't ever be a "perfect time" to take care of your health. The best time to start your health journey was years ago. The second best time is right now. Choose "day one" over "one day."

Action point: Counter trigger the "I'll do it tomorrow" with "Can I do this right now"? The answer is a resounding, "Yes. Yes you can."

DAY 19: EXCUSE-PROOFING PART 2: THE FALSE DICHOTOMY LOOPHOLE

"I can't eat well or train because I'm too busy with _____"

Bull ROAR!

One of our brain's neat little deceptions is to think in binary terms. We tend to hyperfocus on the here and now—of which healthy eating and exercise don't always take center stage in the performance known as life. Life will keep you on your toes. There will always be a steady stream of work deadlines, kid commitments, family obligations and a plethora of unknowns/unpredictables. There will be times where you have less time, where you are more tired and less motivated. These are the times where you double down. Fight to maintain your fitness and health. Scrounge for every opportunity to move and have a healthy meal. Calibrate your expectations, do your best and just do. Do whatever it is in that moment where you can be productive.

Showing up is 90% of the battle. 20 minutes is better than 0 minutes... you CAN make the time for healthy eating—even when you're crazy busy!

-No time for a 5k run? Go for a quick 10 minute walk or run.
-No time to get to the gym? Do squats and push-ups at home.
-No time for a full grocery shop? Just grab a few healthy essentials to make your dinner with.

Remember your priorities. Remember your health has to come first.. Or at least 1b or 1c (alongside family/friends).

> Action point: Focus on what you can do in any given moment. Use the above strategies when you feel in a pinch for time. Always examine and re-examine your priorities.

DAY 20: EXCUSE-PROOFING PART 3: THE "YOLO/FOMO" FALLACY

You only live once! Seize the donut!

Of course you do... and of course you shouldn't deny yourself all culinary pleasures in life. However...

Living life to its fullest CAN and ideally should be accomplished by moderating yummy food. YOLO can (and ideally should) also be applied to the long term health and vitality of your body. Enjoy foods... all foods—but enjoy them in smaller amounts than you are used to... because you choose to, not because you feel you HAVE to. Repeat the message to yourself that you can live life to its fullest without your belly being its fullest.

Many tempting foods and drinks are served at social events, prompting one to Carpe Diem all over a pastry, a plate of fries or every bite of a multi-course brunch. Remind yourself of your long-term plan. Remind yourself that your life will be just fine if you don't partake in this right now. If you choose to, try sampling as much as possible. Cake? Help yourself to a small piece. Cookie? Have one and then walk away... FAR away. Delicious restaurant meal? Take some to go.

If you are in a social situation, try focusing on the company—you are there to enjoy friends/family/coworkers. Yes, food might be a big part of that event/occasion but cognitively lessen its overall importance. Reframe these situations as opportunities to catch up and engage in great conversations rather than opportunities to overindulge. Pick your spots—enjoy 1-2 things that look amazing. My client and good friend Anna has a nifty personal strategy when it comes to indulgent foods: It has to be a 9 or 10/10. That is, if it isn't (or doesn't look like) it would be one of the best desserts you've ever tasted, it's not worth the calories. Why waste calories on a food you are only moderately interested in?

Action Point: Condition yourself to believe that you can enjoy a wonderful existence without having to indulge in every culinary experience you face. Pre-commit to indulgences (the what and how much) beforehand and execute.

DAY 21: EXCUSE-PROOFING PART 4: THE "TODAY IS A SPECIAL DAY" EXCUSE

I'll be blunt here: any day can become a "special" day if we rationalize it to be. Far too often we fall into the trap of excusing errant eating under the guise of "special circumstances."

The problem is that there is always an "occasion" if we look hard enough. Christmas these days tends to be a 4-6 week gingerbread man/latte/house bombardment—rather than a couple of nights of eating in a surplus. And not to mention the bevy of retirements, baby showers, bar mitzvahs, birthdays and other such celebrations that we partake in.

If we choose to overdo it at every possible occasion we will not get very far when it comes to our health and fat loss goals.

Again, pick your spots. Perhaps you know that there will be 3 celebrations this week. Pick one of those to go a little rogue on your normal eating path. Remember also to focus on the company, the occasion, the conversation—not the food.

By extension, your own personal milestones deserve a non-food related celebration. Remember, there are many non-food related ways to celebrate events. The key here is to detach the automatic impulse to pair a marking of an occasion with food and drink. Much of the time, food cannot (nor should it be) avoided, in which case you can move towards the healthiest foods possible under the given circumstances. Have cake on your birthday—100% and consider not having cake every time someone in your workplace of 50 has a birthday (which will be often).

Action Point: Pick your spots. If there's a particular special event where you know there will be amazing food, choose that occasion to indulge. Conversely, know which events you will not partake in.

DAY 22: AVOID THE "CLEAR AND PREDICTABLE PATH" TRAP

When we make plans for the future, we seldom plan for distractions. We assume a perfect-world scenario, free of distractions and diversions. Our clients are no different when they first come to us. They are convinced that they've got this because motivation and discipline won't be problems.

In Marshall Goldsmith's book *Triggers* he notes that in our day to day lives there is a high probability of low probability events. We don't plan for low probability events because they are just that—under the radar and unlikely to happen. However, the odds of at least one of these many events occurring is high.

-*"I had planned on working out but have a work deadline."*
-*"I was going to get some food but my toilet clogged and had to deal with that."*
-*"I was housebound with a sick child home from school."*
-*"Had a blown tire which took half the day to deal with."*
-*"My friend needed an urgent favor."*

The above scenarios aren't common, however the chance of any one of those things happening is far more common than we think.

I recall my first gym job many years ago having a conversation with one of my (particularly jacked) co-workers about how he stayed so fit.

"I don't ever plan a day off," he said.

Seeing the incredulous look on my face he clarified, "Don't get me wrong, I have days off.. but these are unplanned days off when life gets unpredictable."

Enthusiasm for your journey is great, but be honest about the road ahead. Familiarize yourself with the idea that there will be distractions and derailments. With consistent and persistent habits, tending to more urgent life events won't pull you off-track. Do what you can under the circumstance and get right back at your excellent health habits when unpredictable events hit—which they will.

Action Point: Plan something health-progressing daily. Life will throw these at you without your help. Keeping things consistently healthy when life is more predictable will hold you over when things get chaotic.

DAY 23: RELAPSE PLANNING: YOU WILL MESS UP. GET OVER IT QUICKLY (BUT LEARN FROM IT)

Having a strong plan for when you lapse may be one of the single most effective ways of keeping on track over the long haul. A lot of this is grounded in squashing what is known as the "What the hell" effect or as it's called in scientific circles "counter regulatory eating." This is an all-too familiar pattern whereby we eat something we know isn't conducive to our goals. We don't stop there, however—we continue to spiral and continue to overeat because, "Ah, what the hell—I've already blown my diet." One cookie turns into one sleeve of cookies which can turn into half a bag of cookies.

Here is a handy 3-step process to preventing a full blown relapse:

Self-forgiveness: It happened, it was delicious, forgive yourself. This is huge—keep practicing this (I mean, don't deliberately go off plan to get "practice" but when it DOES happen, practice self-kindness).

Self-reflection: What prompted the lapse? Poor planning, stress, social pressure? Figure out what precipitated the event and make a conscious effort to be better prepared next time temptation strikes.

Back at it... immediately: This is crucial. As soon as it happens, make your next meal a healthy one, get to the gym the very next day, put the pieces into place to make your next several meals healthy ones.

Through practice and building habits and the right mindset, lapses will be less frequent and last shorter periods of time. You won't be perfect—and that's ok, but you WILL be more than good enough to make progress.

Hit the reset button—as many times as necessary. Your journey will be a bumpy one. Guaranteed. Your long-term success hinges on your ability to take lapses in stride. Forgive yourself, get back on your path right away and learn from it.

Author James Clear has what he calls a "never miss twice" policy. If you've goofed up, don't goof up twice in a row. Missed a workout? fight like absolute hell to get one in the next day. Had a greasy meal last night after 4 cold ones? Get your groggy butt to the grocery store and get some produce the next day.

Action Point: When things go off track, fight like heck to get back on track right away. Forgive yourself, move on and learn from it.

One of the most impacting books I've read in the area of entrepreneurship is called *The One Thing* by Gary Keller and Jay Papasan. As the title might imply, the theme of the book is focusing on one thing—one task, one project, one objective that will get you to where you want to be in an efficient, effective way. The question they ask of their readers is this,

"What's the ONE thing I could do, such that by doing it everything else would be easier or unnecessary?"

As you may have already guessed, this applies equally to your health pursuits as it does to business pursuits. A unifying theme of the book is that purpose + priority = productivity.

Live with purpose and you'll know where you want to go.
Live by priority and you'll know what to do to get there.

When we wake up everyday we can ask ourselves, "What shall I do?" or "What should I do?" When your life is on purpose, living by priority takes preference. It's about doing the "should do's" over the "want to's" more often than not.

Purpose has the power to shape our lives only in direct proportion to the power of the priority we connect it to. Purpose without priority is powerless. The word is "priority", not "prioritIES." To have a healthy purpose is awesome—that's why you are here. But is your health TRULY a priority? Are you intentionally moving in the direction of better health through your daily actions? If not, focus on what you can do right now to move towards aligning purpose and priority.

Action Point: Shift your focus on what matters most. Always know your next health play, whether that is a brisk walk, a quick healthy meal, chopping veggies, or doing a set of 25 air squats. Always know your purpose, always know what the priority is. Write down 3 immediate actions you can take to keep your priority and purpose in mind.

I feel like in today's social media-centric world and aesthetically-driven culture, we've lost our way when it comes to the concept of "motivation." For one thing, we overvalue its importance and for another, we are looking in the wrong places for its sustained impact.

We are conditioned to derive our motivation from extrinsic sources: outcome goals such as losing weight, being a certain size or achieving a particular look. The research on motivation is becoming more and more clear: extrinsically motivated rewards such as money, status, titles (and yes, a certain weight or body fat percentage) are neither fulfilling nor sustainable. This is what has been termed a "carrot and stick" approach.

Intrinsic rewards, by contrast, are those rewards that come from within—the innate desire to relish in the process. Intrinsic motivation is closely connected to self-determination theory—a framework of motivation and personality proposed by behavioral scientists Richard Ryan and Edward Deci.

SDT focuses on how social and cultural factors can both facilitate or undermine people's sense of initiative and praises the importance of individuals:
- Autonomy
- Competence
- Relatedness

Intrinsic motivation is tightly bound to these principles as we humans tend to be more motivated by having autonomy—a sense of control when it comes to a journey or process.

Even young people have a desire for something more than a tangible reward. When children were asked to paint something and then offered money to paint other works of art, they lost interest. When the children didn't expect a reward, receiving one had little impact on their intrinsic motivation. Only contingent rewards—if you do this, then you'll get that—had the negative effect. Why? These rewards required them to forfeit some of their autonomy.

The key then, is to hone in on the intrinsic aspects of motivation; eating healthily and exercising for the sake of it—for how it makes us feel. You may never LOVE exercise or broccoli. That's ok too! The goal is to internalize the experience and know that it is bringing you closer to who you are meant to be (remember you are meant to be healthy).

Daniel Pink's book *Drive* explains the new frontiers of motivation as having 3 essential elements:

1. Autonomy—the desire to direct our own lives;
2. Mastery—the urge to get better and better at something that matters; and
3. Purpose—the yearning to do what we do in the service of something larger than ourselves.

Finding Flow

A "flow state" is one where a person performing an activity is fully immersed in a feeling of energized focus, full involvement, and enjoyment in the process of the activity. The master of "flow," Mihaly Csikszentmihalyi has this to say about it:

"Most important, in flow, the relationship between what a person had to do and what he could do was perfect. The challenge wasn't too easy. Nor was it too difficult. It was a notch or two beyond his current abilities, which stretched the body and mind in a way that made the effort itself the most delicious reward. That balance produced a degree of focus and satisfaction that easily surpassed other, more quotidian, experiences."

Achieving some purpose and mastery over your tasks involves setting up what are called "Goldilocks" challenges—not too hard, not too easy—nutrition and fitness tasks that will challenge you enough to keep you interested (and progressing) and not too insurmountable that you will be apt to give up. This is what's called an "autotelic" experience—the Greek translation being an end or purpose of itself. The closer we can connect the means and end as one, the more likely we are to become intrinsically motivated.

Losing 10 lbs, fitting into a dress size, etc. are great goals, but if they are not anchored in enjoying the process—training and eating for how it makes you feel—long term success is unlikely.

Pay attention to how you WANT to feel. Enjoy the challenge—embrace the discomfort. Find joy in the accomplishments. This is a journey... a process.

This isn't an easy feat by any means. It may be that you never love going to the gym or that you never quite acquire a taste for peppers, oatmeal or chicken that hasn't been deep fried. If this is you, I suggest attaching your process to what it's doing to your body, more so than how you are feeling.

When engaging in a task that is uncomfortable, think about how your body is being made healthier, the texture of the food, the sensation of your legs as they climb a mountain or do a final set of squats. Embrace these sensations. Take them in and reframe the discomfort as progress—things happening in your body that are taking it to greater levels of health. Pay attention to how you want to feel and keep yourself in that moment.

Motivation is not delivered from a stage nor will it come from motivational posters and memes.

Action Point: How do you want to feel when you exercise? What is a health-enhancing task you can take on that is challenging enough to spark meaningful results, yet not too overwhelming?

If you find yourself struggling to build a good habit or break a bad one, it's not because you have lost your ability to improve. It is often because you have not yet hit that cusp—that point where your nutrition, training and lifestyle changes begin to move the needle —whether that "needle" is literally the one on the scale or the metaphorical needle of progress you have envisioned. James Clear calls this the "Plateau of Latent Potential." He illustrates this point with the story of the stonecutter.

The stonecutter will hammer away at a rock. A hundred strikes later nothing has happened. But the 101st strike will crack a stone in two. It wasn't the last blow that did it, but the hundred before it. None of the effort you have put in already is wasted. Be cognizant about staying focused on your habits and not going on prolonged binges and inactivity, but know that your work was not in vain. Even if you have rebounded from a weight perspective, lost strength or cardio, you will be able to get those attributes back faster.

The work you have put in was not wasted, it was just being stored. If for whatever reason you took a break from your fitness routine, rest assured your brain/muscle connections have a base to go from. Even if you've blown your eating for a few weeks, you have put wiring into place and have equipped yourself with some skills already.

From an observational standpoint, it's not uncommon for me to see people who are seemingly doing all the right things without seeing any physical results and then, inexplicably the needle begins to move. In fact, several times clients have told me they were on the verge of giving up when finally things began to happen.

The work you put in now will never go to waste. Ever. Even if you gain weight back, lose strength, suffer an injury or suffer from a health condition—the work you put is cumulative—especially from a psychological perspective as you've "been there and done this" before and gosh darn it, you can do it again!

Action Point: If you've been putting in the work and haven't seen commensurate results remember that great health dividends are happening at a microscopic level that you can't see. Keep going. Keep charging forward, keep engaging in healthy habits and consider taking a slightly more intense approach from an eating or training perspective. Consider: Is there anywhere else you might be able to scale back food-wise? An extra indulgence you may not have accounted for? Can you bump up your intentional exercise?

Self-awareness is, without a doubt, the most crucial prerequisite to self-discipline—which of course begets continuous results. At the center of self-awareness is the concept of mindfulness; which is essentially defined as a state of active, open attention on the present where you observe your thoughts and feelings from a distance, without judging them as good or bad.

Noted psychiatrist, neurobiologist and mindfulness advocate Dr. Jud Brewer says: *"Mindfulness is just about being really interested in getting close and personal with what's actually going on in our bodies and minds. A willingness to turn towards our experiences—rather than trying to suppress them. It's about approaching our demons with curiosity—which is naturally rewarding."*

In fact, there is some solid research showing the benefits of mindfulness and meditation from a weight loss perspective. In the review of 19 studies, interventions based on mindfulness proved "moderately effective for weight loss" and "largely effective in reducing obesity-related eating behaviors." Interestingly enough, when compared to the "lifestyle change" programs, the mindfulness/meditation intervention had longer lasting results long term. These practices are likely effective due to the heightened awareness around food, triggers and awareness of hunger and fullness.

Further, a 2014 review of 14 studies found that using mindful meditation was an effective intervention for reducing binge eating and emotional eating. The stress-lowering effects of mindfulness meditation can have psychological benefits which can manifest into physical benefits from an inflammation and hormonal response standpoint.

If you are new to this concept like I am, dedicate even a few daily minutes to the practice. One of the misconceptions about mindfulness and meditation is that you should be completely clear of any thoughts while trying to practice. In the early going especially, you may find your mind is abuzz with activity—What will I wear to that work presentation I need to give...who's getting the kids to piano this week...I can't believe Taylor Swift just released another album already.. Didn't she just release a new one last week?! Focus first on slowing down the breathing. Bring a sense of calm over your body as best you can. Get into a quiet, electronic-free, distraction-free place and just sit—on the floor, in a chair, on a bed—doesn't matter.

Here's a simple "mindfulness for noobs" exercise you can partake in, which only takes a few minutes.

-Sit in a chair in a quiet room with your eyes closed

-Don't worry too much about your breathing rate/depth but notice it.. Notice the inhalation and exhalation. Notice the structures around your breathing.. Your shoulders, your ribcage, your chest. Notice how they move with each breath.

-Begin thinking about your feet. Feel the sensation of them on the ground. Move up to your knees, your hips, your abdomen and circle back to the breathing.

Eventually you will be able to do this for longer stretches of time. Taking a step outside yourself and looking at your situation through a non-judgemental lens, taking time in silence and thoughtful reflection can reap some powerful benefits when it comes to making better health and life decisions.

Here are a couple of techniques that I have found to be personally effective in diverting from these negative emotions: "surfing the urge" and "leaves on a stream." These are grounded in the science known as acceptance and commitment therapy.

Surfing the Urge

Urge surfing is a technique developed by Sarah Bowen and Alan Marlatt. This method can be used to avoid acting on any behavior that you want to reduce or stop. In this case we are talking about overeating and staying sedentary but it could be rage, impulse shopping, pornography, drinking or smoking. Here are some things to equip you for surfing the urges.

-Urges are short-lived: Rarely do urges last longer than 30 minutes if we don't feed them. Do your best not to dwell on them, give them attention or justify acting on them. They will feel intense and perpetual in the moment but they will run their course.

-Suppressing a thought, feeling or sensation ultimately increases it. Fighting urges (even by trying to talk yourself out of them or distracting from them) often makes them bigger.

-You can't get rid of urges. You can, however practice ways to accept them and ride the proverbial wave out without giving in to them.

Here are some mindfulness techniques to help you surf the urge:

-Pay attention to your breathing. Don't alter it. Let the breath do its work—slowly.

-Notice your thoughts and without judging, feeding or fighting your thoughts, gently bring your attention back to the breath.

This cognitive defusion exercise, developed by Dr. Russel Harris involves visualizing yourself sitting beside a gently flowing stream with leaves floating along the surface of the water.

-For a few minutes, take each thought that enters your mind and place it on a leaf... let it float by. Do this with each thought—pleasurable, painful, or neutral. Even if you have joyous or enthusiastic thoughts, place them on a leaf and let them float by.

-If your thoughts momentarily stop, continue to watch the stream. Sooner or later, your thoughts will start up again.

-Allow the stream to flow at its own pace. Don't try to speed it up and rush your thoughts along. You're not trying to rush the leaves along or "get rid" of your thoughts. You are allowing them to come and go at their own pace.

If your mind starts to wonder and thoughts like, "This is dumb," or "I'm bored," start to creep in, place those thoughts on leaves, too. If a leaf gets stuck, allow it to hang around until it's ready to float by.

Action Point: Schedule 5 minutes today to practice Leaves on the Stream. If you face an urge you don't want to act on today, give yourself an opportunity to practice Surfing the Urge.

While food quantity and quality is of utmost importance, your relationship with food is even more paramount. You may have to change the way you look at food as a whole. Many people have a dysfunctional relationship or a love/hate relationship with food. Our culture has done an exceptional job of instilling unnecessary fear into the vulnerable psyches of those who are desperate to lose weight. Our fad-loving, pop diet book society has lionized and demonized foods—creating dichotomy and confusion at every turn. We are exposed to maple syrup cleanses, egg-only regimens, carbophobia, fat phobia and yes, the hottest new trend at the time of this writing is Keto's inbred cousin, the "Carnivore diet" (*because fruits and vegetables are clearly responsible for obesity and poor digestive health*).

Part of my job is to help you view food and eating through a different lens. Help you develop a personal philosophy that is flexible, effective and ultimately allows you to make peace with food.

My preferred 3 healthy ways to look at food are as follows:

- Relaxed

- Neutral

- Augmenting

Looking at food as the ally and your nourishment will promote reframing of eating and help guide you towards not only making healthier choices, but nurturing a healthier relationship around food. The goal here is to reduce anxiety associated with food choices.

Next time you eat healthier food—think about how you are being fueled. When you eat foods lower in nutrients and higher in calories, do so in a relaxed and non-judgemental way.

What I'm advocating for, ultimately is food freedom. Food freedom is a 2-way street; releasing from the perceived need to consume certain foods, whilst being forgiving if you do consume said food. In other words, enjoy the freedom and control you have to exercise some restraint; the freedom to say, "No, thank you, I'm choosing NOT to have this right now." When you do happen to indulge in a way that is counter to your goals, there is a freedom in self-forgiveness—in saying, "Yep, I ate more than I had planned and that's ok, it was delicious and I'm moving on."

I won't pretend this is an easy mindset switch. This may take a while to minimize the cycle of feeling out of control and the subsequent self-blame and guilt.

Action Point: Remember, food is neutral, food is fueling and food choices are not linked to morality. You are someone who is choosing more nutrient dense foods most of the time and someone who chooses to eat something indulgent once in a while and chooses not to feel guilty about it.

In any given moment our drive to eat may be driven by emotions. (Remember the bit about us humans not being logical?) More specifically, our emotions can often lead to overeating high calorie/low nutrient foods. Triggers come in many forms and can be categorized into internal and external sources. Internal triggers are emotions and feelings such as:

- Inadequacy

- Insecurities

- Pessimism

- Unrealistic expectations

- Self-defeatist thinking

External triggers are people, places and things:

- Major life changes

- Work

- Family

Regardless of the source, in any given moment of any day you may be feeling one or a combination of the following:

- Stress/anxiety

- Loneliness

- Anger

- Sadness/depression/hopelessness

- Boredom

The problem is that these emotions become part of a routine—an automatic response from your brain. The key here is to disrupt this trigger-to-action cycle.

Emotions vs Emotional Sensations

Dr. Jeffery Schwartz in his book *You Are Not Your Brain* stresses that we need to recognize the difference between emotions and emotional sensations. Emotions are real, genuine and should be valued and taken seriously. Emotional sensations, on the other hand, are false messages—tricks, deceptions and ploys to pull you off-track. These are to be ignored, re-framed and cast aside.

In Marshall Goldsmith's book, *Triggers* he proposes there is a 5 sequence event of behavior; Trigger, impulse, awareness, choice, behavior.

The space between the trigger and behavior is a short but crucial window. Do whatever you can to interrupt the middle. Create that disruptive voice—the "stop" mechanism... again you are asking questions, throwing a wrench in your internal subconscious mechanisms that are pushing you in an unhelpful direction.

Here are some other ways to disrupt this cycle.

Practice Eating Mindfully

Fully immerse yourself in the process of eating. Eat slowly, notice the aroma, the texture, the sound it makes, the temperature, the color and of course, the taste of the food. Pay attention to how your body is experiencing the food. Where in the body are you sensing hunger?

Where is the satisfaction coming from? Consume it deliberately, methodically and without judgement. Practice this for at least one meal every other day—particularly if it's a rich meal.

Seek out Distractions and Alternatives

If you are finding food the only thing that comforts you, I invite you to take a deep look at some constructive alternatives. And look, I promise not to be that sanctimonious jerk that tells you to just do burpees instead of eating a delicious cookie. What I will suggest is other pleasurable activities that can give you the similar dopamine pleasure center-tickling sensations.

Draw a bubble bath

Call a friend—pretend like it's the olden days (pre-2004)

Brew a nice berry tea or a sugar-free cup of cocoa

Crack open a good page-turner of a novel

Listen to some music—fire up your own personal "chill" or "hype-up" playlist.

And maybe, just maybe you might be inclined to do something intentionally active. Jump on that inkling right away.

Build Tolerance to Difficult Feelings

This may sound counterintuitive as we have an inborn human tendency to avoid negative emotions. Let yourself feel anger, sadness, and stress in doses. In fact, embrace them if you can.

Reframe them as signals that something needs attention. Just remember to ask yourself if they are real, genuine emotions or emotional sensations.

Don't Forget the Physiology

While emotions imply a psychological state, there are physical factors at play—primarily related to keeping yourself satisfactorily nourished. Be sure you are eating at intervals that are not leaving you hungry in vulnerable times. It is harder to overeat if you are not hungry. Here are some examples of common scenarios that often trigger unhealthy action with some reflective responses:

Situation: Early afternoon at work and fatigue has set in. Your immediate response is to grab a coffee and a donut at the work cafeteria.

The trigger: You're tired, you may be stressed or anxious, as well.
Ask yourself: Are you truly hungry? Is a coffee and a donut really the best solution? Is there a sound alternative? What if you have just a coffee—black or with just milk or cream? If you are truly hungry, you will find a healthier option in the cafeteria.

Situation: You're home on a Saturday night. You're addicted to this show and you usually raid the fridge or order in while you binge watch.
The trigger: Alone on Saturday night. You're feeling lazy, a bit lonely and maybe a bit sad, too.
Ask yourself: "Am I truly hungry right now or am I doing this out of routine? Is there a healthier option here already? Can I watch my show and find a better option for dinner? Can I go to the grocery store and pick something up that will be fast and reasonably healthy.

Situation: You've had a fight with a significant other and you're left angry. Your first thought is, "I need to have something sweet."
The trigger: Anger due to something your partner said.
Ask yourself: Is turning to sweet food the solution here or is there a better way to deal with this negative emotion? What if I just go for a brisk walk, call a friend or listen to some music instead?

If you feel you are struggling with perpetual cycles of emotional eating, binge eating or otherwise unhealthy food-related behaviors I do recommend talking to a counselor who specializes in this field. Getting the help you need is a brave and virtuous step in getting yourself on a path towards health.

Action Point: 1. Practice mindful eating on one of your next meals. Integrate it into your regular routine of eating.
 2. Draw from your list of alternative pleasurable, yet non-destructive activities when faced with temptation or potential temptation.

PART 2: BETTER HABITS FOR FAT LOSS

DAY 30: IT'S ALL ABOUT HABITS

Your success in health and more broadly, in life will largely boil down to habits. Habits aren't a piece of your journey—they are monumental. One study suggested that 40% of what we do on a day-to-day basis is grounded in habits (it's worth noting that this estimate has been challenged but needless to say, habits are still important). Habits are the brain's autopilot. Our habits are what we repeatedly do and repeatedly expose ourselves to. We are, in essence a sum total of our habits.

The problem with habits is that.. well.. they're hard. Like really hard. We have deeply rooted instincts and patterns that remain intact from our ancient ancestors. Our brains were designed in a time when the best way to save was to consume. As mentioned early on, we now have a perfect storm of ancient, consume-first/consume-often wiring in a modern society with an abundance of hyper-palatable food and technology. In his groundbreaking book, *Atomic Habits*, James Clear describes our habits as "modern day solutions to ancient desires." So much of our behavior is dependent on how we interpret events that happen to us—rather than the objective reality thereof.

As mentioned before, we are irrational beings that run largely on emotion. In any given moment we are responding to triggers and conditioning of given situations—much of which is subconscious. A craving, for example is a sense that something is missing—an urgent desire to change your internal state. Binge eating, drinking and social media consumption isn't about the donuts, the craft beer or the "likes" and positive comments—it's about regulating your feelings. It's about bridging the gap between how you currently feel and how you want to feel. Eventually, our brains begin to equate social media with validation, YouTube and video gaming as escapes and mutual matches as an instant security-booster. Our brains will steer us towards these things to bring us comfort. Just about all human behavior is motivated by a desire to escape discomfort, according to the prolific behavior and tech blogger Nir Eyal, author of the books *Hooked* and *Indistractable*.

So much of this journey has to do with recognizing and quickly managing triggers—bringing previously subconscious thoughts into our conscious radar.

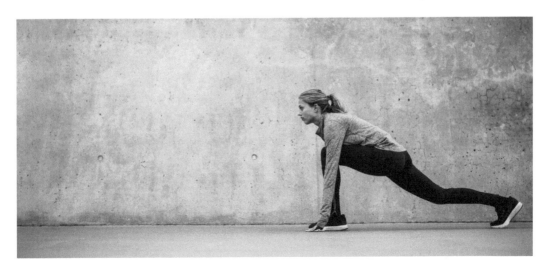

Creating new habits is, in essence, changing our brain's wiring. When we take action, the brain fires to forge new pathways—new neural connections. The concept is known as "Hebb's Law" and basically states that what fires together, wires together. In other words, the more we expose ourselves to various actions, the stronger those neural connections become. Those old, bumpy dirt roads of our brain connections become smoothly paved highways. Conversely, what UN-fires together, UN-wires together. Hence, we can disrupt unhelpful habits by taking different action to break those neural pathways that have kept us in an undesired state. Meaningful change requires both the formation of new, productive habits and the minimization of the disruptive habits.

Action Point: Develop an awareness of your habits. Start thinking about certain patterns that you follow daily. You can do this by journaling-write everything down that you do in a day. Log a couple of days worth of activities. See if you can detect patterns that might be pulling you off track.

DAY 31: CREATING HABITS REQUIRES A FORCEFUL RE-DIRECT

Habits are tricky beasts. Our brains wire to our actions—to what we do on a day-in, day-out basis. As mentioned, our brain establishes comfort zones and directs our behavior towards those comforts—whether it is food, video gaming, online shopping or nail-biting. Our brains perceive change as a threat. Overriding this will require a fight. Our brain wires itself to what we do—habits emerge from repeated actions and is shaped by what we expose ourselves to. Our brain doesn't have a moral compass. It doesn't know a good habit from a bad one. The biggest challenge is to change how we respond to emotions. It will take a great, repeated force to find different coping mechanisms.

- This is going to be challenging
- This is going to take belligerent consistency
- It is going to take uncomfortable action. It gets easier.
- Habit development is not linear; you will have an easier time on some days than others
- You will never be free from temptations, urges, or the lure of habits that pull you away from your goals.
- Habit formation takes longer than you think it will.

How many days does it take for a habit to take hold? If you go by conventional wisdom, you are likely thinking 21.

More rigorous research, however, confirms that it is more like 66 days (on average) to form a habit. Three times longer than most of us have been taught to believe. This of course depends on many factors (type and stronghold of the habit as well as genetic and environmental factors) but for a particularly sticky habit, prepare yourself for a couple of months of consistency for it to solidify. It may take more days, it may take fewer days, but what it will take is laser focused regularity. The problem is that most people give up way before they allow a habit to stick. Making a habit stick takes more time than most of us are comfortable with.

While 66 provides a rough average, habit formation is more about the repetition and exposure than it is the number of days.

Action Point: Pick one habit. Put 100% of your mental/emotional/physical resources into that ONE habit. Whether it's not having a donut before work or a drink after work, or going on a fast food run at lunch or having a snack at night, find a single habit you want to break and go after it. For 2 full months. This is how long it may take for your brain to un-wire this habit.

It's time to flip the script. Use the internal dialogue. Say no to emotional sensations or say yes to better responses. When in doubt go back to Day 7 and just act.

In the simplest terms possible, for a habit to stick you have to make it as easy as possible. We have to appeal to our lizard brains and our propensities for warm couches. We need to find the laziest way possible to maximize our habits for things to stick. The best ways to make habits easy are to:

1. Engineer your environment

We are going to unpack this concept in a multi-part series to follow. I will say that shaping your environment is without a doubt one of the most important strategies for forming habits. Making better habits easier through environmental nudges will reduce the cognitive load and the need to conjure up willpower. This WILL be one of the most important points of this book so I thought I'd plant the seed now.

2. Reduce Choice

We live in a world of abundant choice. Consider the average supermarket carries in excess of 42,000 items. Through food delivery services we can have most restaurant fare at our doorsteps. We have become the unwilling victims of a psychological force called the "paradox of choice," often leading to "analysis paralysis."

This paradox of choice theory—coined by psychologist Barry Schwartz, posits that our vast options when it comes to modern life—whether choosing food, TV shows, school courses or a potential mate on a dating app are doing more harm than good. They are interfering with our ability to manage time and make concrete decisions. The better we can eliminate the mental load of decision-making, the easier it becomes to focus on things that matter. To wit, the average woman spends 15 minutes per day choosing what to wear—this can account for a full 190 days worth of staring at a closet over a lifetime. You may have heard of a handful of highly successful people who wear the same clothes daily to reduce this cognitive backlog.

Countering these forces through strategic de-cluttering will give us the clarity to make our health pursuits much easier. Here's a list of ways you can avert choice paralysis to make better health decisions.

- Reduce choices in as many aspects of your life as you can. Focus on only designating mental resources to important choice.
- Breakfast is the one meal where people don't mind as much having more limited options. Have 1-3 breakfast options and put them on rotation.
- Pick 3-4 staple meals to eat on a weekly basis. Consider setting aside a day for a specific type of dish, such as meatless Monday, turkey Tuesday (ok, taco Tuesday), chicken Thursday, fish Friday.

- Do 1 exercise program at a time. By all means, mix up your variables and types of training (cardio, strength) but see one program through for a good 4 weeks at least before switching.
- Grocery shop from a limited and specific list (more on grocery shopping savvy to come).

3. Automate whenever possible

A few short years ago, the organ donation rate in Austria was 99%. In Germany it was 12%. How is it that in such similar cultures there is such a vast discrepancy? Are the Austrian's far more noble citizens than their German counterparts? Nein. The difference is in the opt-in versus opt-out systems in the respective nations. Austrians had to fill out paperwork to opt out of donating their organs whereas the Germans had fill out paperwork to opt IN. This made it easier for an entire nation to donate their organs in the event of a tragedy.

Locking into company benefit plans help people invest, automated deposits into savings accounts help people save. The same types of strategies can be employed to easily boost your health. These are what behavior experts call "commitment devices."

Here are some ways you can lock habits into place to simplify your health journey:
- Automate a grocery store delivery on a weekly basis. Many grocery stores both deliver and gather your goods for easy pickup.
- Use a meal delivery service on days where you know you will be too tired to cook.
- Use push notifications to alert you when it's time to hit the weights, meditate or start your slow cooker.
- Join a class or sports league, committing yourself into 1-2 active sessions per week.- Hire a personal trainer: Having an appointment weekly (or 2-3 times weekly) will help ensure those are not only active but supervised/guided.

4. Shape the Path

The key here is to take the easiest possible step to get healthy food into your pie hole and intentional movement into your day.

- Put shoes on, go outside.
- Join a gym that is VERY convenient and show up there at least 3 times a week.
- Put a mat and some weights down in front of your TV.
- Buy a roasted chicken and some veggies and an already cooked sweet potato at the grocery store.
- Chop one pepper.

> **Action Point:** Put effort into simplification. Remember that your brain and your body will always choose the path of least resistance. Instead of trying to fight a tendency to conserve, work WITH your brain and implement easier, plug-and-play solutions. Start thinking about how to make things easier targets.

- A long run feel daunting? Put your shoes on.
- An hour long slog in the gym too much? Get on the floor and do a few squats, push-ups and some ab work.
- Is cooking an elaborate meal making your brain hurt? Grab a roasted chicken, some frozen veggies and pre-made grains.

Don't take this the wrong way but I'm going to ask you to stop dreaming. That's right, cast aside your fitness and health fantasies, your perfect "beach body," your butt that you can bounce quarters off of. I get it, it's far more alluring to think about jaws dropping as you slowly walk into your high school reunion wearing that sleeveless dress showing your ripped arms. It's appealing to think about walking slowly out of the shallow waters of the ocean like Daniel Craig in his first Bond movie—revealing your chiseled abs in a slightly too small pair of blue swimming trunks. I think we are all guilty of a little fantasy when it comes to envisioning our "best selves" and this is normal and, to a small extent, useful. I am here to assure you that what appears to be me stomping on your dreams is for the greater good. Let me explain this from yet another chapter in the giant book called *"your brain is kind of a dick."*

The problem with this ideology is that our brains don't do a very good job of separating fantasy from reality. In our minds we have already created a delusion of achievement and it dulls the "action orientation" centers of the brain. In short, the whole "experience your success as if it has already materialized" is a fast track to nowhere.

Psychology professor Gabriele Oettengen has spent much of her career turning conventional pop psychology on its head. From Stuart Smalley-like mantras (cueing all 90's Saturday Night Live fans—"I'm good enough, I'm smart enough and dog-gone it, people like me")— to the runaway cult classic The Secret, we've been taught that we need to believe it, picture it, manifest it—yadda, yadda... well turns out that is mostly a steaming pile of nonsense.

Perhaps the most glaring misgivings about big dreams is that they prompt "big steps," which almost always results in failure. What I'm advocating here is what Sean D. Young, author of the excellent book *Stick With It* calls the "stepladder" approach. Accumulating incremental, small wins and building upon them—or "chaining" them together one link at a time.

What we are doing here is leveraging our brain's desire for more instant gratification— gaming the "current moment bias" or "delay discounting" tendencies of our reactive and pleasure-seeking brains. By chaining together smaller, quick hit type of rewards in the form of small wins, we are leveraging a crucial neurotransmitter called dopamine. Dopamine isn't so much a "pleasure" entity as it is an "anticipation of pleasure" process.

According to Young, our brains understand reward in relative, not absolute terms. For example, dopamine is released if someone is expecting a small or medium reward and gets a medium reward. If someone is expecting a medium or LARGE reward however, and gets the medium reward—no dopamine is released and there is a subsequent letdown. As will be explained later, this is a huge reason why focusing less on outcome goals is beneficial.

I'll give you a few common examples on how to modify goals to optimize the chaining effect using very common anchoring points in the realm of nutrition and fitness.

1. Instead of aiming for 10,000 daily steps, record a week's worth of step counts and divide by 7 to find the average. Set a goal of increasing this average by 1000 steps.
2. Instead of targeting for 1g per pound of body weight in protein, track how much you take in on average and aim to bolster it by 20g/day.
3. 5 servings of veggies is a fantastic goal...if you currently eat 3-4 servings per day. If, however, you only have 1, aim for 2-3.

These small, incremental changes will keep building. Focus on the readily attainable and don't look back.

> **Action Point:** Pick something you already do that is good for your health and set a target to increase it by a small, easily achievable amount.

DAY 34: INTRIGUING: MAKE YOUR JOURNEY COMPELLING

For any habit to take shape, you'll have to find a way to enjoy it—or at the very least not hate it. While you may rarely initially feel like putting the work in, you can and should make the process as smooth, intriguing and joyful as humanly possible.

Author and professor Ian Bogost has a fascinating take deriving pleasure from tasks that are not prototypically pleasurable. He advises detaching from what we think fun "should" feel like. The attractiveness becomes the effect of what you're doing, not to cause. Again we see the importance of reframing—in this case we are reframing difficult work as "fun." The fun becomes the challenge, the striving, the embracing of the suck.

Here are a few ways to look at making your health journey compelling.

1. Game-ify your Health

Now if you are a gamer, I'm not going to try and convince you that eating more broccoli and knocking out 3 heavy sets of lunges has comparable appeal to "Fortnight." What I am saying is reframe your tasks so that you see your health pursuits as a game—a winnable game. Video games remain compelling even though there is an 80% failure rate of finishing. Take delight and find some exhilaration in the pursuit and the challenge. Like video games, your healthy lifestyle takes practice and bit by bit you become better at it. Can you go that extra mile per hour on the treadmill? Can you go that extra mile on your run? Can you do squats for a minute straight? Can you bench press half your body weight 10 times? Set these challenges up and see them as games—always on the lookout for a new achievement.

And yes many apps exist that can help add an element of fun and "game-ification" to your workouts and health. Some of the more popular ones are:

- -Zombie runs
- -Burn Your Fat With Me
- -Superhero Workouts

2. Temptation Bundle

Temptation bundling is a term coined by behavior specialist and Wharton School professor Katy Milkman—a noted leader in the field of helping people make better decisions. This technique involves taking something you enjoy and pairing it with something you should do (i.e. workout or prepare healthy snacks). In a landmark study she authored in 2013 entitled "Holding the Hunger Games Hostage at the Gym: An Evaluation of Temptation Bundling" (I would have picked a much less crappy film as an example, but you get the idea),

Milkman showed that participants who were instructed they could only listen to audiobooks while at the gym were 51% more likely show up at the gym than the control group. Here are a few examples of temptation bundling:

- Watch a TV show on a stationary bike. If there is a series you like or if you watch the news, ensure you watch it while on a piece of cardio equipment. Ditto, of course, with the above study using an audiobook or a podcast.
- Put together a great playlist before a strength workout to get into the "zone."
- You can use the audiobook/podcast TV show idea when you chop veggies or prepare a meal, too.

3. Engage the Power of Grown-up Play

For most of us, the end of childhood also signals the end of the instinct to simply "play." Children innately gravitate towards spontaneous activity and play regardless of the situation. The only thing stopping us from continuing to play into adulthood (within reason) is our own perceptions.

This again comes down to prompting, inserting a trigger or an antecedent. It's about implanting the instinct to play with your kids or nieces and nephews whenever possible (active play and games). Make use of parks, open fields, open spaces, your living room. With children everything looks like a playground. Within reason try and frame things this way. Climb stairs as fast as you can, bear crawl or crab walk. Do pull-ups on bars if you can.

4. Add Novelty

While I believe in repeating basics and mastering a few key habits rather than chasing variety, I like the idea of adding something different to a workout or food prep that can give things a bit of a boost. Trying different recipes, different spices, different healthy restaurants can break up the monotony. Trying a different class or a different movement at the gym can give that little extra motivator you might need that day. I work a lot with young people who struggle with weight and activity. I like to get them on the rowing ergometer and have them play "the fish game" where they have to row away from the big fish and eat the little ones. You can do this even as a grown up!

5. Reward the right way

Rewards can be a slippery slope but when done right they can work well. We spoke earlier about intrinsic motivation—the reward being the process itself. This is of course ideal—that the reward IS the habit—the hard work, the journey; how your lifestyle makes you feel, your results, your sense of accomplishment. Those should be the bedrock of how you perceive "rewards."

While you may never "feel" like doing something initially, you may surprise yourself in how great it feels when you're in it. My goal isn't to try to convert you into one of those annoying "clean eating, always-working-out and posting about it on Instagram" types of people; rather, I'm inviting you to see if you can derive some joy out of this process and maybe, just maybe, challenge yourself to have a bit of fun while doing it.

A productive reward might be something along the lines of putting money into a travel fund or an item you like. Open a separate account and stash money in there that would have been spent on a meal out or for reaching a predetermined weight or health goal.

Action Point: What are your opportunities to make your health journey more compelling? Download a gamification app to help shake things up and/or set up a "fun fund" in a bank account and put into it when you reach goals.

The entire end game of habits is that they become permanently etched into your brain's wiring, where it becomes almost unconscious, to a point where things will feel "off" if you somehow did not partake. I know that after not exercising for even a couple of days I get irritable and even have physical symptoms like feeling stiff, weak and achy. Ditto if I've been eating off plan—low energy, irritated gut and just plain uninspired.

Making habits part of your brain mapping involves a repeated, deliberate action in the direction of the healthy habits. Putting these actions into play involves the previous 3 pillars of habit change: making them easy, chaining them and making them compelling.

The brain is complex and efficient. It stores things that frequently occur so that it can be easily accessed—our brains want to relax and attain a homeostasis. Here are some methods to help anagrammatically lock-in habits.

1. Repeat the same behaviors—same time, same place

Whatever new habit you are trying to adopt, set things up in a way that you can do so in a consistent time and place. This starts with a consistent sleep/wake-up time. Even on weekends, I recommend keeping your sleep times relatively similar to your weekday times. Whether you bike, gym or go to classes, try hitting these on the same times/days whenever possible. Ditto with grocery shopping, taking supplements and other non-physical health-related habits.

2. Meditation/Mindfulness session

Having a daily mindfulness or meditation session will go a long way in helping develop patience by changing the brain mapping. Meditation and mindfulness can increase awareness, improve concentration and retrain the brain for new psychological responses. It can lead to lasting changes in health via this new structural wiring.

3. Deploy the habit stacking and temptation bundling

Habit associations will help routine-ize your healthy intentions. Associate waiting for the coffee to brew with putting healthy snacks in a bag, a podcast goes well with your meal prep, an episode of your favorite 44 minute TV drama pairs nicely with a stationary bike.

The Power of Starting rituals

Professional athletes are well known for their pre-game/pre-race rituals, ranging from logical movement preparation-type exercises to bordering-on-bizarre antics (hockey goalies that talk to their goalposts). Many athletes swear by these rituals and are convinced that they play a role in how well they perform.

And while these rituals do not impact the chance nature of bounces or increased speeds in a race, studies have shown that these routines strengthen feelings of control and confidence that may otherwise be lacking. This increase in self-efficacy is what can have application to those of us who don't make millions of dollars to perform.

The application to us regular folks is the value of ingraining habits. Charles Duhigg's *Power of Habits* argues the virtues of "personal starting rituals" to battle procrastination. He notes,

"One way to use habits to fight procrastination is to develop a habitualized response to starting. When people talk about procrastination, what they're usually talking about is the first step. In general, if people can habitualize that first step, it makes it a lot easier."

We can create our own "pre-game" rituals to prompt us for action. My favorite go-to is playing a "hype up" song mix—something a bit jarring that gets me into a workout mode. If I'm prepping for making a healthy meal, it may be a podcast or a more low key indie playlist. Just getting on the floor and doing a mobility circuit can get you into the right headspace to crush a strength workout. You can also use non-related rituals. It could be brewing and drinking a cup of coffee, making a bed or reading a Bible verse or from a book of quotes.

Rituals can not only help you kickstart healthier habits but they make the actual habit more enriching. They can make food taste better and believe it or not, proposing a toast makes the drink taste better (really).

Harvard professor Francesca Gino and colleagues tested the power of rituals in trying to get people to eat less. One half of the participants were told to be mindful about their food consumption for the next five days. The other half were instructed to undergo a three-step pre-eating ritual and were advised to complete it every time they ate something. The ritual involved:

- Cutting food into pieces
- Rearranging the pieces so they were perfectly symmetrical on the plate
- Pressing the eating utensils against the top of their food 3 times.

Participants who enacted the pre-eating ritual consumed fewer calories (about 1,424 calories for each day, on average) as compared to those who simply were mindful about their eating (who consumed about 1,648)—a 16% difference. The ritual group also ate less fat and less sugar. The ritual helped them with the self-control needed to achieve their weight loss goals.

Gino found similar results with participants faced with carrots and chocolate—with 58% of those in the ritual group choosing carrots over chocolate vs. 35% of the control group.

So while tapping your food 3 times with your fork may not be your go-to ritual (I would have to recommend against it on a first date), there are some things that you can do to help ritualize your food consumption.

-Say grace or give some kind of thanks before meals.
-Take in the aroma of the food for a minute before digging in—enjoying the fragrance (if there is one associated with this meal).
-Take a sip of water first.

A fringe benefit of ingraining habits is that when life throws that inevitable curveball and you are forced off the wagon, it is easier to re-engage from a brain wiring/habits perspective. From a food standpoint it could mean getting back into meal prep and healthy eating. From a training standpoint, you have neuromuscular connections already in place that will help get your strength and stamina back faster than if you had been sedentary.

Action Point: Develop a starting ritual for your meal preparation and training sessions. What are the easiest habits you can lock into place starting today?

Preparation is the centerpiece to healthy eating and it starts in the grocery store. No habit will help better prepare you for healthy eating than consistent grocery store shopping, chopping and preparation. Making the time for this "holy trinity" of fat loss habits is essential. I understand, life gets hectic. We tend to wait until we open the fridge, stare at the sad, wilting produce and several bottles of dressing, condiments, the last of the milk and realize, "Dang it, we need groceries, but I'll do it tomorrow and order something tonight."

Grocery Store Zen

The modern supermarket is designed to get you to buy a lot of food and to buy especially a lot of the high profit-margin foods. These are the foods that tend not to be good for us. Grocery stores often smell like baked goods deliciousness and subtly entice us in those directions. Here are some concise strategies on grocery shopping like a boss:

- The first step is to make grocery shopping a sacred 1-2x/week habit. Have a consistent day or 2 during the week where you grocery shop, chop and prepare your food. I find Sunday is a logical day to do a big shop (if you aren't working on Sunday).
- Pick another day where you can pick up extra produce or things you may run out of.
- Shop from a prepared list. Do not stray from this list and do not add anything to the list that will derail your healthy eating habits.
- Your prepared list should include staple healthy items, ingredients for a couple of recipes and some "on-the-go/emergency" items. (see below)

- Don't shop while hungry and yes there will be impulsive temptations there (baked goods, chocolate, ice cream, etc). Walk right by them. Stick to the list!
- Perimeter shop for most of your items; this is where the produce, meats/meat alternatives are. When in the aisles, think canned goods, spices, nuts/seeds.
- Use your grocery store in lieu of a fast food place—particularly one that has a "hot food, meals-on-the-go" section (ensure that your on-the-go meals here are not of the deep fried variety)

Solid grocery shopping should accomplish 3 things;

1. Build a solid kitchen inventory.
2. Provide needed ingredients for a week's worth of healthy meals.
3. Fail-proof an on-the-go lifestyle through healthy, convenient snacking.

Keep this process simple. Your grocery store experience is what will set you up for easier, healthy eats.

STAPLES/RECIPE STUFF	HEALTHY CONVENIENCE
Protein: poultry, beef, fish, eggs, tofu, edamame, seitan	In-a-pinch, need a quick meal: • Roasted chicken • Pre-cooked beef strips • Hard boiled eggs • Frozen veggies • Pre-cut/washed greens/veggies • Baby carrots • Frozen, healthy(ish) meals: (look for higher protein, lower calorie, veggie-filled brands. • Also frozen burritos, frozen chicken or fish can be an option.
Vegetables: leafy greens, peppers, cucumbers, tomatoes, broccoli, cauliflower, carrots—basically any vegetables you like. Frozen veggies.	
Fruits: Berries especially but apples, bananas and other fruits you like. (frozen fruit is good too)	
Dairy or dairy substitute: milk, nut milk, soy milk), plain greek yogurt, cottage cheese, cheese, oatmeal.	Portable • Small tuna cans/packets (flavored) • Beef/turkey/salmon/soy jerky • Mixed nuts • Seeds (pumpkin, sunflower) • Dried chickpeas • High protein commercially-produced snack
Canned goods: Tomato sauce, tuna, pumpkin puree, beans/lentils.	
Dry goods: Whole grains/quinoa	
Spices: Garlic/ginger, oils/vinegars, olive oil, soup base, stock	Portable/desperate Protein bar (low sugar)
High fiber: High fiber tortillas, high fiber cereal (more than 4g fiber, less than 5g sugar).	

Now that you have a framework for grocery store savviness, let's get to step 2: The chopping/prepping.

Basically as soon as you get home, chop up anything that requires it. Get into the habit of making several servings worth of something (i.e. cook several chicken breasts, prepare a large one-pot meal, chop veggies so you can easily make a salad). If you have a barbecue, take full advantage and use the entire surface area of the grill.

Next comes the prepping. Again we are going to make this as simple as humanly possible. Think about your typical days and think about how you can easily and healthily fuel yourself.

What you'll need are containers of various sizes—try not to skimp on quality here as you will be using them often.

Start small and start with making a LOT more food than you'll need for dinner—this is the easiest way to meal prep. This way you can just portion things out for a couple more healthy meals for lunches.

Single pot meals are the easiest thing to start with. A stew, casserole or thick soup can work well.

The components of a good meal prep kit are:

- Protein
- Veggie
- High fiber carb

There are plenty of resources on easy meal prep strategies online. Just type in "high protein, easy meal prep."

Essentially, don't leave your place without having at least 3 healthy things. This could look something like this:

- Leftovers
- Apple
- Can of tuna
- Baby carrots

A good grocery shopping and food prep rhythm takes time to master but once you get some traction it becomes easier. Just get used to wiring yourself towards going in the fridge and taking something healthy with you, or chopping some veggies or marinating some chicken or tofu.

Action Point: Find some simple, healthy, higher protein recipes and write down the ingredients. Plan your next grocery shop and set aside time for chopping, preparation and portioning.

DAY 37: THE PAUSE/BREATHE/REFLECT METHOD FOR AVERTING DIET DISASTERS

I've adapted this universally helpful strategy from psychology and behavior expert Kelly McGonigal from her excellent book *The Willpower Instinct*. I've expanded what she terms the "pause and plan response" to the "pause/breathe/reflect method." This strategy is immediately deployable under a variety of circumstances and is especially useful in the face of temptation.

The very act of just stopping yourself for a moment allows you to breathe. When you breathe, breathe slowly (about 4 breaths a minute). For an explanation of the importance of slowing the breathing down, I will briefly explain the concept of heart rate variability (HRV).

Here's a mercifully brief explanation about HRV. Everybody's heart rate varies to some degree. In a healthy heart, there are normal fluctuations—your heart speeds up a bit when you inhale and slows down again when you exhale—all normal stuff. In a stressful situation, however, the sympathetic nervous system takes command, spiking the heart rate up and lowering the variability, locking the heart rate into a faster state. This fuels feelings of anxiety or anger. In contrast, when we slow down the breathing and reclaim self-control, the parasympathetic nervous system takes over to calm stress and quell impulsive actions. Heart rate goes down, but variability goes up. There are studies to back up its positive effect on heart rate regulation.

And guess what else slow breathing and high HRV is associated with? Willpower and self-control. Slowing down our breathing gives us mental clarity and basically allows the logical sides of our brains more opportunities to make sensible decisions.

Pausing first allows for slow breathing which makes way for reflection. While you are slowing your breathing down, reflect on what's in front of you. Whether you are facing a plate of fresh cookies, the desire to skip out on your workout or feel the impulse to yell at your kids or a co-worker—reflect on the long-term goals and remind yourself that you are in control.

I can't emphasize this enough... use the pause, breathe, reflect method early and often. The goal is for this to become a reflexive response to stress and temptation and to help you master any situation.

Use this strategy over and over until it becomes habitual to make mindful and informed decisions when it comes to food.

Action Point: Practice this right now—slow your breathing down. Let your mind relax. The next time you are faced with a tempting high calorie indulgence, go right into pausing, deep breathing and reflecting. Is this something you really need right now? Is there a better alternative? Are you truly hungry or responding to an emotional sensation?

Charles Duhigg's book, *The Power of Habit*, outlines what he calls "habit loops"—a 3 step series of events that forms the genesis of most habits. These consist of a cue, a routine and a reward.

Cue: The cue is essentially a trigger. The cue can manifest itself in different ways; it could be a time, a location, a situation, other people, an emotional state or an immediately preceding action.

Routine: This is the habit that follows the cue—the potentially undesirable habit pulling you away from productivity, goals and progress. It could be a morning frappuccino, late night snacking, smoking or mindless social media scrolling.

Reward: The reward is what makes doing the routine worthwhile—according to our brain. The problem is that what our brain perceives as a reward might not be very good for you long-term (remember our ancient wiring and its bias for the immediate).

To understand your own habits, Duhigg suggests you identify the components of your loops. Once you have diagnosed the habit loop of a particular behavior, you can look for ways to displace old vices with new routines.

What's the cue for your undesirable routine? Is it hunger? Boredom? fatigue? The need for a break?

And what's the reward? The donut itself? The change of scenery? The temporary distraction? Socializing? Or the burst of energy from the sugar rush?

What normally precedes your poor eating habits or your diversion from exercise? How can you change the routine and still derive a reward from it?

For example, do you make a daily trip to a coffee shop on the way to work? (cue). Normally get a muffin with your coffee? (routine).

Feel satisfied by the muffin (reward). Flip the script. Go to the coffee shop and get your coffee (sugar free). Either skip the muffin or opt for something healthier (some cafes have protein boxes, for instance, but you will have brought your boiled egg, spoonful of tuna, olives and cherry tomatoes from home. Right?. Same cue, similar reward (caffeine...mmm) but different routine.

Find the simplest path possible here. The best method is something I will expand on later called an "implementation intention." (Day 41). This is simply making an advance plan—knowing your triggers in advance and how you will respond to said triggers.

To give you a case study, I'll draw an example of a young client of mine (early 20's). He had been in a cycle of overeating, especially in restaurants that he would frequent. His cue was simply a drive to eat—a physiological hunger and the impulse to go to his favorite restaurant, a barbecue place where you fill a bowl with a variety of foods and someone cooks it. His routine was to fill two bowls to be cooked. I asked if he would be open to trying just one bowl and putting more filling protein and veggies in it. He agreed and when he tried it out, he wasn't left hungry and still derived the reward of feeling satisfied with a much lower caloric hit.

Action Point: Ask yourself how you can still obtain a reward with a different routine. What are your alternatives? Start today—look at a habit you are struggling with. How can you interrupt the routine to improve your health?

Habits are the compound interest of self-improvement—yet another gem I learned from James Clear. The effect of your habits multiply as you repeat them. One of the problems is that we don't see immediate payoffs of our healthy habits. A few days of healthy eating, 4 times at the gym this week, saying no to donuts at the office on Thursday; none of these will put a noticeable dent in our progress in a week or two yet the impact they have over several months or over a year can be astounding.

The reverse is also true. We don't see a burger and fries meal out as a big deal (nor should we), because we don't see an immediate spike in our pant sizes, nor will skipping the gym negate all of our "gainz." The cumulative effect, however of 2-3 fast food meals out and missing 1-2 gym sessions a week over time will have long term consequences.

In short, a 1% difference either way will have an enormous compound effect long-term. If you've had a great streak going but are frustrated about the lack of physical manifestation of results... relax.

Keep focused. Keep going. Keep fighting. If you've blown off the gym and had a few more meals out than usual—don't beat yourself up, but do get back at it right away.

Success is the product of daily habits. Resist the urge to let impatience and discouragement over what you perceive to be a lack of noticeable results throw you off course. Keep striving for better, keep chipping away, keep aiming for a 1% improvement, keep hitting singles. Remember the chaining of habits—use the stepladders.

> **Action Point:** What is one small thing you can add and one small thing you can take away so that you will make incremental steps towards your goals? It could be an earlier bedtime, bringing food to work 3 out of 5 days, eating out one less time during the week. Pick 1-2.

Habits very often form and piggyback from other habits—sometimes in a good way, oftentimes not. One of the easiest yet effective ways to build healthy habits is to stack them onto another habit.

The key to consistency is to treat a habit stack like a single action instead of a series of individual tasks—this will make new habits seem less overwhelming. In his book *Habit Stacking* etc, S.J. Scott outlines some crucial steps on how to implement these stacks to benefit every important aspect of your existence. Here are some steps to executing habit stacks:

1. Start in small time frames: I advise starting small here, 3-10 minutes ideally. This draws on the concept of keeping things as ridiculously easy as possible. Later I will discuss breaking your habits down into 5- minute blocks of time.
2. Focus on small wins: Remember from the lesson in chaining—create an atmosphere where you collect small wins. Pick the easiest habit to change. This could be a weigh-in, filling a water bottle, doing one yoga pose or a brief breathing exercise.
3. Pick a time and location: Every habit stack should be tethered to a specific time and location. Here are some examples:
   - Upon waking: Great routines can start as soon as you get out of bed. We will expand on some "starting rituals" and "keystone habits" later but think about how you can set yourself up for a healthy day through a couple of strategic moves.
   - Morning (work): Water bottle at desk, healthy food in reach.
   - Lunch: Healthy options from home or healthier meal out, take a walk, mindfulness/meditation.
   - After work: Drive straight to the gym, straight home or to a grocery store for healthier food options.
   - At night: Engage in a hobby, family time, listening to music, going for a walk, doing a few yoga poses, making a cup of tea.

4. Anchor your habit stack to an existing trigger: A trigger should be an existing habit—something you already do on a daily basis like brushing your teeth, showering, making coffee, putting on your seatbelt, etc.
5. Create a checklist: This list should include the sequence of the intended actions, how long it takes to complete each one, and where you'll do them.

Put the above on a repeat rotation and watch as new habits form and become your new normal. Here is an example of what you can do from a health enhancement standpoint through habit stacking:

CURRENT HABIT		STACK WITH
Upon walking	→	Glass of water
Coffee brewing	→	Preapare/Pack 3 healthy snacks/lunch
Brushing teeth	→	Squat (dynamic or held)
At work (lunch)	→	Walk around outside/protein
On your way home	→	Grocery store (if needed)/gym
Dinner prep	→	Water/push-ups/chop veggies
TV show/movie	→	Stationary bike/treadmill
Bedtime	→	Plan next days meal/reflect

Action Point: Design your own personalized habit stack. Pick 3 from the above list or come up with your own that are more customized to your needs.

DAY 41: IMPLEMENTATION INTENTIONS

This is simply a fancy, science-y sounding term for a "plan." Implementation intentions are one of the most useful daily tools you can have in your arsenal of habits. This entails mapping out in your mind how you will ensure a healthy day. Think about this the night before and as soon as you wake up. It is basically inserting an "if/then" trigger into your psyche to enhance follow-through. If you are anything like me, you might spend a lot of your life "winging it"— operating on unfulfilled good intentions. What helps is applying specifics to our intentions. A "which day/what time, where and how" needs to be applied to the "what" of our intentions. This bolsters the chances of your habit taking form.

An intriguing study demonstrated the impact of setting implementation intentions from the British Journal of Health Psychology. Study participants were placed into 3 groups:

The first group was the control group. They were simply asked to track how often they exercised.

The second group was the "motivation" group. They were asked not only to track their workouts but also to read some material on the benefits of exercise. The group was also educated on how exercise could reduce the risk of coronary heart disease and improve heart health.

The third group received the same presentation as the second group, which ensured that they had equal levels of motivation. This difference in this group, however, is that they were also asked to furnish a plan for when and where they would exercise over the following week. Specifically, each member of the third group completed the following sentence: "During the next week, I will partake in at least 20 minutes of vigorous exercise on [DAY] at [TIME] in [PLACE]."

The results were pretty hard to ignore. At follow up the researchers examined how many in each group exercised at least 1x per week. The results were as follows:

Control Group: 38%
Motivation Group: 35%
Intention Group: 91%

This both underscores the importance of implementation intentions as well as the reduced importance of "motivation" (notice this group actually fared WORSE than the control group). Implementation intentions are also a particularly useful strategy when there is an event/holiday or any social situation where there will be access to rich food.

Wake up every morning thinking, "What can I do today to be healthy?" then plot out the specifics. We will cover these aspects more in the goal setting mastery section but let's take a look at a few examples of how we can draw out intentions.

One of the most effective strategies is to follow the "WOOP" method (Wish, Outcome, Obstacle, Plan). In the meantime, here are a couple of examples on how to set up and follow-through with intentions:

- -Monday, 7am: Back, Legs + 15 min hard cardio on rower and treadmill at my gym.
- -Tuesday: 7:30pm: Grocery store run: Pick up chicken, mixed veggies, eggs, chickpeas, quinoa, almond milk, mixed berries from grocery store near work. Return home at 8:15 and marinate chicken, chop veggies and cook a batch for dinner and next days lunch.
- -Thursday upon waking: Mindfulness/meditation before checking phone

> **Action Point:** Create your implementation intentions for this week with food and training. Be sure to include the what, when (day and time), where and how (if applicable).

DAY 42: ENVIRONMENT MASTERY: NUDGING AND CHOICE ARCHITECTURE

As alluded to before, motivation, willpower and sheer passion are overrated when it comes to achievement. Engineering an environment in a way that we are less reliant on willpower, however works wonders. Configuring your environment is one of the most effective ways of leveraging the "simplify to optimize" principle we talked about on day 32. By optimizing your environment you are making habits easier to accomplish.

Richard Thaler and Cass Sunstein wrote a groundbreaking book called *Nudge*. A nudge is a subtle, often tiny coaxing in the direction towards a desirable action. It is a harbinger of shaping the environment and the basis of what they call "choice architecture" (a title I use to describe what I do as a coach). By setting up an environment in which we are "nudged" into a productive action, we can subconsciously (and hence easily) spark ourselves into action and form the building blocks of habits. These nudges have been used by governments, corporations, small businesses and individuals alike to direct behaviors.

There are some fascinating sociological experiments in which nudging has produced some impressive results. Some of which include:

- Using a cardboard cutout of a security guard to reduce everything from speeding to bagel theft.
- Using a picture of a real handicapped person instead of the generic symbol to reduce incidences of people parking in handicap spots.
- Painting a mural of Hindu Gods in an alley to prevent people from urinating on the walls (while we're on the topic of peeing)
- Putting a moving target on urinals prevented men from peeing on the floor (I seriously wonder what's wrong with my gender sometimes)
- Putting a second bowl of guac out with a "double dippers only" post-it on it just about eliminated double dipping heathens.
- Strategically placed nudges and environmental architecture can produce some substantial results when it comes to making healthy changes.

Perhaps one of the most striking global examples of environment shaping behavior is in the study of "blue zones"—areas of the world with the highest concentration of healthy centenarians (100+ year olds) on the planet (Ikaria, Greece; Okinawa, Japan; Sardinia; Loma Linda, California; and Nicoya, Costa Rica). Longevity expert and bestselling author Dan Buettner made a remarkable discovery when studying these blue zones; their physical environment was ideally designed for health-enhancing behaviors.

For example:

Terrain: Blue zone-ers lived in mountainous and otherwise challenging to traverse landscapes making both getting around and importing processed goods a giant pain in the butt.

Home and Office Design: In places like Okinawa, Japan, chairs are harder to come by, which makes for more walking. Sardinian homes are vertically oriented which forces a lot of stair climbing. The close physical proximity of these buildings also contributes to more neighborly interaction, increasing the community feel and strengthening social connections.

Peer Influence: Taking rest times once a week is important in many of these communities. They make time for friends, family, exercise and cooking fresh food. There is a social contagion at work here as citizens old and young level to what the norm is.

Now it may not be in the cards for you to move to one of these blue zones so you will have to work backwards to create the most health-centric environment possible.

Action Point: Here are a few easy-to-get-started actions for mastering your environment:

1. Make desirable habits 20 seconds easier and undesirable ones 20 seconds harder;
2. When setting up your personal world for success, think about how you can reduce friction on accomplishing tasks and how you can increase friction on things you want to avoid. Keep a water bottle within arms reach and the candy bowl well out of arm's reach.
3. Task association: Have one place at your home where you eat (preferably a table, not a couch while watching TV).
4. Review the habit loop/habit stacking strategies and keep implementing them.

There are 3 primary environments that you will have to tackle to make your healthier habits smoother:

1. Your home
2. Your workplace/commute
3. Your social time

The environment over which we have the most control is our home. Go into your kitchen. I'm going to ask you to shake up your kitchen in such a way to make it as convenient as possible to eat healthfully while making it as inconvenient as possible to eat poorly.

This starts in the grocery store and I cannot even begin to emphasize how important your grocery shopping is (more on this later). For right now I want you to buy into the gospel of "out of sight, out of mind… in sight, in mind… in hand, in mouth." What does this mean?

Store healthy food front and center

Whether on your countertop, in cupboards, in your fridge or freezer, keep healthy food at eye level, in plain sight and in see-through containers. These foods should be yelling "EAT ME" every time you open the fridge, a pantry cupboard door or look at your countertop.

Keep least healthy foods out of the house

Don't bring them into your house. If you have to get off the couch, put pants on (stupid laws and societal norms), get in your car and drive to your nearest corner store to indulge in KitKat ice cream you will be much less likely to actually follow through than if the treat is a mere 14 steps away in your freezer.

Keep less healthy foods in the back of cupboards

If you do happen to have empty calorie foods in the house, put them in the furthest reaches of the fridge or cupboard. Make these foods hard to access.

Use smaller plates and bowls

For all the recent controversy of Brian Wansink's research methods and validity, there is no denying that eating off of smaller plates and out of smaller bowls with smaller utensils is conducive to eating less.

Keep your gym bag at your door and athletic shoes in plain sight

You should have to trip over these items to get outside.

Keep exercise implements in a room you go to often

I keep my foam roller and a set of kettlebells on my apartment floor as I know it's the only way I will use them.

> Action Point: Put some of these things into place TODAY. Place healthy things where you will see them and consume them.

DAY 44: ENVIRONMENTAL MASTERY PART 2: THE OFFICE/COMMUTE

Take a lot of what you apply to your home environment into your work environment. Because many of us spend a great deal of time commuting and working away from home, our travel and work environments are vital to set-up to ensure we keep healthy habits humming along.

Pack lunches and snacks daily
Don't leave your home without at least three healthy items. Grab an apple or another portable fruit, higher protein snacks like hard boiled eggs, jerky, cheese string, baby carrots or a low sugar protein bar.

Prep your car for hunger pangs
Have a car inventory with an emergency snack or two (nuts, seeds, beef jerky, low sugar protein bar, small can of tuna). Keep plastic utensils and wet naps in the glove compartment.

At work, stay as far away from unhealthy options as possible.
You will statistically halve your chances of consuming candy if it is in a jar a few meters away than if it is on your own desk. What should you have on your own desk (aside from a picture of loved ones and a voodoo doll of your boss with a book entitled *Voodoo for Dummies*)?

A water bottle and some healthy snacks, like cut up veggies, fruit or any of the items listed as part of your car inventory.

Hit the grocery store instead of the fast food joints
Get used to doing a quick shop at the grocery store, rather than what may have been a pattern of drive thrus. It doesn't take much longer to do a quick run for healthier food and the health benefits will accumulate substantially over time.

Move your body
Make it a habit to get up and move around if you sit at a desk for much of the day. From a general physical and mental health standpoint, getting outside and walking around—even if only for 5-10 minutes—can reap significant benefits.

Action Point: Set your work environment up so that you can stay healthy while away from home. Water bottle and healthy meals and snacks front and center.

DAY 45: ENVIRONMENTAL MASTERY PART 3: YOUR SOCIAL ENVIRONMENT

In the words of noted psychologist and author Roy Baumeister, "social distance matters more than physical distance when it comes to food." If you are a particularly sociable person this will apply to you a little more. Social environment in this sense is both the physical environment (restaurant or house party) as well as the company you keep.

Here's what you can do to navigate social situations:

Hang around more fit people

People who value being fit will be better role models and influences in your eating and activity decisions. Weight has a social contagion effect. While those who live in blue zones are part of a social norm of activity and healthy eating, those who hang with people who engage in less healthy behaviors take on those behaviors. The Framingham Heart study showed that if your 3 best friends are overweight—your chances of becoming overweight increases by 57%.

Suggest more active or healthy outings

Why not organize walks/hikes/bike rides? Local trampoline park, laser tag, a group fitness class? You might even be able to combine sedentary, food-based outings with some activity ie. post dinner walk, picnic (weather permitting). Maybe even throw out the idea of a healthy potluck? Give everyone a chance to sample healthy yet tasty foods.

Remember your pre-commitment

Have fun but have your pre-commitment plan in place. Recall the if/then concept (if I'm offered desserts I will say "looks delicious but no thank you"). Your plan might be to go for higher protein and veggies, whole foods or a small portion of dessert or a single glass of alcohol. Customize it to the situation.

I understand that there is social/peer pressure to let loose and "come on, have a drink, relax" or "you HAVE to try this dessert... and this one, too." People who are being indulgent feel better when others are too and will try and rope you into indulging with them. Remember; YOU are in control, you are on a path, you get to make these decisions.

Sometimes it helps to text people in advance and let them know you are challenging yourself to adopt healthier habits. You can also up the ante by letting them know you will pay them $20 if they catch you ordering more than 1 drink, eating dessert or (insert indulgence here). I will speak more to this in the following day (loss aversion).

So, absolutely enjoy social outings. Enjoy those "fun" friends who love to eat and drink. Choose, however, to partake in a way that aligns with your goals, your vision and most importantly—your identity. And who knows, maybe you'll inspire friends and family members to adopt a healthier lifestyle with you.

When it comes to dining out, I like a few simple guidelines:

1. Skip the bread (I know it's warm, I know it's delicious, I know you're very hungry)
2. Drink water only (or a glass of wine...maybe 2...MAYBE).
3. Take some of the meal to go. Seriously, this is a perfectly reasonable and effective way to cut back on the number of calories consumed by spreading a single meal over 2.
4. Order something with a good chunk of protein and opt for salad (dressing on the side) instead of fries.

Work diligently on creating a social climate that is conducive to progress. Control what you can and remember that YOU are in control. Absolutely, 100%, enjoy some indulgences and let loose a bit. Do, however stay focused on aligning with who you are, not who you used to be. Enjoy the actual social aspect of the situation—focus on the company, the conversation and make food and drink the secondary part of the event.

When your significant other isn't on board

This is a common scenario and presents a very real obstacle for progress. Your significant other may be resistant to change himself (usually men here—sorry, guys) and even resistant to your change. Here are a few things to keep in mind as you move forward with the person you love by your side much of the time:

-Remember that your significant other and others that live with you may not be ready for change. Talk to them about it, let them know you would really appreciate their help, let them know specifically HOW they can help you and thank them in advance.

-You may have to take on more responsibility for the cooking if you don't already.

-If you are the one who typically buys the groceries, don't buy junk food. If someone in your house wants something specific, have them get it themselves and instruct them to hide it from you.

-Communicate some mutual "rules." For instance, promise not to bug your significant other about changing his/her ways and in return ask your significant other not to eat their unhealthy snacks in front of you.

-Encourage, nudge, role model and tell them how great you feel since you've changed your eating habits. Do not, however, judge them or nag them to eat more healthfully.

-With friends, try and plan active get-togethers where you are walking instead of going for a meal. If you go out, remember to make and follow through with your implementation intention.

-Commit to fewer social events. I'm a big believer in finding a happy medium.. For example, if you are used to going out for drinks 2-3 nights after work and then once on the weekend, consider shaving this down to 1 weeknight, 1 weekend. Then, when out you still employ your implementation intentions. Perhaps you only order 1 drink and an appetizer that is greens or protein-based.

-Limit time with unhelpful friends. In some circumstances I don't think it's out of the question to choose not to hang out with certain people. Now far be it from me to suggest we should ditch friends because they aren't as helpful to our lifestyles, however, if you feel that friend is constantly trying to coax you into decisions that pull you off track, that friend may not be a very good friend anyway. Just my opinion—take it for what it's worth.

Action Point: Have a specific plan in place for each night out. Plan your indulgences and stick with that plan. Practice dialogue with friends and significant others that keeps you on track ie. practice saying "looks delicious but not right now, thank you". Have your "if/then" plan ready to roll on every occasion.

We are built to hate losing. Psychologists estimate that losses feel twice as bad as wins feel good. Therefore, we would generally rather avoid losses than catch wins. One interesting technique for changing difficult habits is to employ loss aversion. BUT, there are ways proven effective and ineffective when it comes to this. The right types of incentives, built on a strong foundation of intrinsically motivated and self-determination-based mindset driven approaches, can help bolster change through public declaration and a little extra something.

Stikk.com was formed by Yale Behavioral Economics professor Dean Karlin who was looking for an effective way to follow through with his weight loss goals. Stikk.com leverages loss aversion through a commitment contract. Basically you pick a goal, design parameters and then enlist a referee, as well as some stakes.

Research conducted by Karlin suggests that having a "referee" (accountability partner) triples your chance of succeeding and having a financial disincentive triples success rates.

The effectiveness of the financial loss is bolstered by having to donate to an "anti-charity." Pick a political party you dislike, a movement you can't stand and pledge that you will donate $100 to that cause if you don't reach your goal. Why it works is because you think about giving your despised political party your hard-earned money when you are faced with a tempting food. This is often enough to help you pause, breathe, and reflect—remember what you learned on Day 37?

You can simply place a friendly bet with a buddy, colleague or significant other as well. But make sure you enlist someone who will hold you accountable. The secret sauce behind this concept is the declaration, the accountability and the courage to "put it out there."

There is a significant mindset/psychological value in the bravery of making your goal public. If you are hesitant about this sort of strategy, ask yourself why. Often this is a combination of a fear of failure and/or a desire to stay comfortable and avoid accountability. Both of these are perfectly understandable, but both perfectly correctable. I do advise a bit of reflection here and taking steps towards eliminating trepidation around accountability and fear of failure.

Action Point: Gather up the courage to make your health goals known to others who will keep you accountable. Put something on the line that will mean something to you. Recruit someone who you feel has excellent self-control and will keep you on track. Offer $20 to an entire group of people if they catch you ordering more than 1 drink or dessert.

Being in motion and taking action are two ideas that sound similar, but there is an important difference. When you're in motion you are planning, strategizing and learning. All great things, BUT being in motion does not produce results. Taking action, on the other hand, is the type of behavior that delivers an outcome. We often default to being in motion because it allows us to feel like we're making progress without running the risk of failure. Motion gives us the illusion of results when really it's the "act now" mentality that really brings results. This is paraphrased from James Clear's book, *Atomic Habits*.

On a personal note, this one resonated with me a lot as I tend to use "planning" i.e. "being in motion" as a proxy for real action. I've read countless books on psychology, entrepreneurship, and sales but when it comes to implementing the strategies therin I've fallen way short. I have enough "ideas" to make myself a multi-millionaire and have read enough books to do a phD dissertation on behavioral economics. When it comes to writing, financial planning even meal prep, however, I've had to stop myself from being in motion and take action.

As soon as you catch yourself "in motion," remind yourself to take deliberate action. Plan your week of meals, yes. Plan your gym schedule, absolutely. But get to the grocery store, come home and chop/cook/prep, go to the gym or get on your weight set in the basement. Planning has its place but it should take FAR less time than the actual action.

Some things to watch for here when it comes to "being in motion":

-Sitting and writing, refining and mulling over a plan.

-Being overly meticulous about details.

-The perception that you can't take action unless _____ happens first.

-Reading too much about how to make yourself better—continuously soaking up information and not acting on said information.

Don't let planning get in the way of your action. You already know enough to make significant health improvements.

Action Point: Insert an action-oriented trigger for when you are tempted to "plan" something as a proxy for action. A grocery list is great, writing down goals is great and planning your weekly intentions is great. Spending time in these activities as a substitute for action won't get you anywhere fast, however. As soon as you feel the urge to seek out more information online or taking out books on the subject, ask "what can I be doing right now that will take me closer to where I want to be?".

Being part of a community and having a strong support network can be very beneficial for keeping on track with your journey. The more people you have behind your efforts, both in person and in the e-world, the better. One of the longest running, most successful weight loss programs in history, "Weight Watchers," modeled their program on this concept.

Having been both a dieting member of a support community, as well as having run a private accountability and support group, I have witnessed the life-changing value of it.

When it comes to online support groups there are benefits in terms of fat loss—provided the participants are engaged and adhering to food journaling and progress recording. It's more likely that those in a social online group are more apt to partake in journaling and progress reports and hence yield better results.

For example, results from Journal of the Royal Society Interface showed that at the six-month point, members who were not social networking had lost an average of 4.1 percent of their body weight. Those with two to nine friends lost an average of 5.2 percent; those in the giant cluster lost 6.8 percent and those with the most exchanges of online communication lost more than 8% of their body weight. This online community accountability works especially well for people with the higher engagements and belief in the process.

In real life, support is even more important. Whether it is from a spouse or other family, friends or co-workers, a strong network of support can be very beneficial. Telling as many people as you can about your goals and specifically how they can help support you, can provide the extra accountability and encouragement you need to stay on course. A great community should be full of encouragement and accountability. Here are some other aspects of communities that provide an environment conducive to thriving.

One that establishes trust
This is a space where you need to feel comfortable to be vulnerable. A place of non-judgement and empathetic ears.

One that is inclusive
A community that welcomes people from all walks of life—different stages of change, different circumstances, different challenges but with a common goal of improving health.

A place of empowerment
A community should empower you and help inspire its members. Interactions should mostly leave people feeling like they can accomplish something.

A place to share wins, struggles and observations about the journey
A well-moderated space where there are people who take the lead in conversations, moderating conversations and ensuring the community runs smoothly and remains a place of growth and support.

You never have to be alone in your journey. There are people just like you out there with struggles like yours who would be comforted to know they are not alone either.

> **Action Point:** Declare and proclaim your intentions to your supportive friends and family in real life. Join one-maybe two online support groups that fit the above criteria with the aim of learning, supporting, asking questions and reporting results. (Note: I encourage minimizing time spent in online support groups as it can detract from taking action).

DAY 49: MASTERY

About 8 years ago I watched a documentary called *Jiro Dreams of Sushi* about a remarkable man named Jiro Ono (94 years old at the time of this publication). Jiro is the proprietor of "Sukiyabashi Jiro" in Tokyo who, for 50 plus years, made the trek to work at his 3 Michelin star restaurant—one of the most celebrated sushi restaurants in the world. The movie depicts Jiro taking painstaking, deliberate measures and rituals in creating the very best sushi in the world.

The Japanese are originators of some very cool, very deep wisdom when it comes to learning, growing, progressing and finding balance—of which mastery plays a big part. I'll focus on 2 concepts here.

Shokunin: The rough translation of this word is "craftsman" or "artisan" but the true meaning goes deeper than this. The Japanese apprentice is taught that shokunin means not only having technical skills, but also implies an attitude and social consciousness.Shokunin is a "mastery of one's profession"—one who is fully devoted to their craft.

Another Japanese concept that resonates with me when it comes to the concept of mastery is "Kaizen"—a term meaning "change for better." Kaizen has found its way into company mission statements, self-help books and performance coaching. The idea of constantly improving, continuously striving for better and forward progress are keystone approaches to mastery.

Mastery is a key component of intrinsic motivation. Mastery is the desire to improve. If you are motivated by mastery, you'll be more likely to see enormous potential within yourself, and you'll constantly look for ways to improve your skills through learning and practice. Previously mentioned author Daniel Pink outlines 3 laws of mastery:

1. **Mastery is a mindset:** This involves a conviction that you CAN improve your current state. That you have an internal locus of control—agency over your situation. It means you know there will be bumps along the way and you will forgive yourself and keep going—no matter what.

2. **Mastery is a pain:** Improvement can and will feel like a grind at times. Those who see success tend to habit-ize the mundane tasks that yield improvement. It's what researcher Daniel Chambliss calls "the mundanity of excellence."

3. **Mastery is simultaneously alluring and frustrating:** It's the realization that you won't ever FULLY master anything, but it is alluring enough that you will keep trying and keep striving for better.

When it comes to eating and training, seek the "Goldilocks" challenges you learned about on Day 25. These are the actions that that will challenge you enough that you feel a sense of accomplishment but not so much that they frustrate you to the point of giving up.

Aim to continuously improve. Decide that you are going to defy the laws of aging, defy the statistics of "normal" age-related decline, belligerently pursue greater strength, stamina, mobility and lower body fat despite having a busy career, social life, family and other commitments. Bask in the thrill and exhilaration of the chasing better and better.

Action Point: Find ways to stretch your comfort zone in a way that furthers your health. Become a better health chef by trying recipes, aim for a new personal best in your squat or deadlift, run a distance you've never run before. Keep working on the most important aspects of your health-keep igniting that internal fire of striving for better.

Whether it's in the self help section of the local bookstore or social media memes, so much is made about "being happy." The "self help" industry has an estimated value of over $10 Billion—with multitudes of books festooning the bookstores with the promise of living a life of perpetual bliss.

You may have seen a widely shared article in 2015 with a very alluring headline "What 75 Years of Happiness Research has Taught us " or "Harvard Study Reveals the Secret to Happiness" or some such variation. As a reminder, here are some of the findings from this study:

- Happiness comes from choosing to be happy with whatever you do, strengthening your closest relationships and taking care of yourself physically, financially and emotionally.

- Happiness evolves from nurturing the 3 "goods:"

1. **Do good for others:** Spend time and energy doing good for others—particularly those less fortunate than you.

2. **Do good for your soul:** Doing things that you have an interest in or that you are good at can make you happier. What are your hobbies? passion projects? Is there a skill that you have been wanting to learn for a while and just never pursued it? Start now. It's never too late to discover new passions or at least try different things—even if you don't end up loving it.

3. **Do good for your health:** Your health is your greatest asset. Live in such a way that you honor your health—giving your body the best in any given imperfect circumstances.

When all the dust settles, most experts agree that happiness really comes down to the strength of our social connections. In fact, an absence of tightly knit relationships is hazardous to your health—shockingly, as much of a risk as smoking and cancer. Draw closer to those you love and whose company you enjoy. Make time for family and friends, engaging with the ones that make you feel heard, valued and loved. Seek out social connection with people who nurture your best self.

Happiness is how we navigate the world around us—framing our circumstances in the most positive way possible. Happiness is feeling fulfilled in our realities. The correlation between happiness and occupation, income or wealth is far less that the correlation between happiness and how people feel about their occupation, income or wealth.

One thing I've noticed over the last 10 years of social media is that we are constantly prodded into being "extraordinary." Personally, I am drawn to the idea of finding the extraordinary in the ordinary.

Constantly striving for some form of superstardom or worldly success detracts from enjoying the present. As Mark Manson says, the vast majority of our lives are spent in the humdrum of day to day life. Keep learning, keep growing, keep progressing--without feeling the external pressures and temptations of viral fame. In other words, be you, only braver.

Happiness and Aging

Atul Gawande's book *Being Mortal* cites the work of Laura Carstensen, PhD researcher on aging who noted that as we age, our general sense of wellbeing actually improves.This phenomenon seems counterintuitive considering the decline of physical capacity as we age. Older people are more satisfied with their social relationships than are younger people, especially regarding relationships with their children and younger relatives.

Older people are generally less prone to anxiety, depression and anger. Carstensen's studies demonstrated unequivocally that as time passed, so too did emotional satisfaction and stability.

This begs the question that if we make gradual shift as we age into greater appreciation of everyday pleasures and relationships, rather than achievement, acquisition and possession, why do we take so long to appreciate it?

The Power of Gratitude

We've probably all heard that we should practice being grateful. What many people don't know, however, is the most effective way to practice gratitude. Simply listing what you are grateful for is, of course, helpful and develops a level of appreciation.

A different, particularly effective technique is called the "George Bailey" method. If you've ever seen the iconic Christmas classic It's a Wonderful Life, you'll recall the angel trying to convince George not to commit suicide by showing him what life would be like for others without him.

I'll ask you to try gratitude practice this way; picture the most important few people in your life right now. Imagine now that they don't exist. Think about the emptiness and deep sadness you would feel without them. This may be temporarily emotionally jarring but this taps deeper into the centers that help us truly appreciate who and what we are grateful for.

I have to say that I am grateful that you have made it this far in the book. Now let's go to where the rubber meets the road and devise a bulletproof plan to take you to where you want to be.

Action Point: Try the "George Bailey" method of gratitude. Picture what your life would be like without those you care about the most and your activities that fill your soul.

GOAL SETTING MASTERY AND GOAL CRUSHING ACTION

Setting goals is the most common, yet skimped on portion of the health transformation journey. Goals provide direction and focus for what we want to accomplish. Typical goal-setting measures, however can be largely incomplete and hence ineffective. There are a few reasons why the typical model of goal-setting is flawed, most notable being that they are conceived of in a moment of utopia, assuming a clear path and a predictable future. They remain static entities with myopic outcomes that tend to lack staying power—usually as a "New Years Resolution" state of optimistic bliss.

The go-to goal-setting acronym is "S.M.A.R.T." (Specific, Measurable, Attainable, Realistic, Time-oriented). All these components provide a solid backbone, but adequate follow-through is necessary. It is important to reframe how we see goals and spend more time in a soul-searching, deep dive through a realistic lens kind of journey. Through many years of helping people work through their goals, I've devised a system that I truly believe can set people up for sustainable success.

Here are my 3 primary pillars of goal-setting mastery.

GOAL SETTING PART 1: FINDING YOUR WHY AND CLAIMING YOUR IDENTITY

What is your "why"? Think about your most profound desires, your "raison d'etre." Simon Sinek popularized the concept of finding your "why" in his excellent book Start with Why: etc and his TED talks that preach similar messages. While goals tend to focus on the "what," the "why" is far more important as it gives the "what" meaning.

Why is your health important to you?

A typical goal-setting session might look like this:

You want to lose 10 lbs in the next 2 months? Excellent. Why?

"Because I want to look better and be healthier."

Why?

"Because I feel better about myself if I'm healthier and will be more confident if I look better."

Why is that important to you?

"I have a wife that I care about and family who count on me."

The above scenario helps guide people towards their deeper and underlying desires that go beyond the outcome goals of scale weight. Think deeply and think from the heart.

Be able to clearly articulate this. It might be the ability to do the things you love well into older age. It may be the ability to play sports with your grandkids. It may be to live independently for as long as possible.

Personally I find my "why" in being an excellent role model for my children. Secondarily, I thoroughly enjoy hiking. I live in one of the hiking meccas of the world in Vancouver, Canada and when I reach the peak of a mountain and take in the stunning views, I often think about wanting to experience this well into old age.

Everyone will have a different "why" and it doesn't necessarily have to be about family or friends but if is helpful to have a profound reason for improving your health.

Your answer to the "miracle" question

This is straight out of the counseling model known as "Solutions-focused Brief Therapy." The miracle question is: If you were to magically wake up tomorrow and you are at your goal (picture the perfect version of you), what is the first thing you would notice? The first thing that would be different about your life?

Again dig deep here. How would you feel, describe what your life would look like.

You: A Pursuer of Optimal Health

Your current behaviors are simply a reflection of your current identity. Rather than trying to chase outcome goals, focus on building and then aligning with an identity. You are not changing your body as much as you are changing WHO you are—your beliefs, your values systems.

Who would be more likely to vote in an election, the person who says "I'm going to vote" or the person who says "I am a voter?" Such a study did take place and predictably, those who identified as voters followed through with voting at a significantly higher rate.

Are you "someone who throws bottles into recycling bin" or are you "a recycler?"
Are you "trying to stay fit and healthy" or are you "a healthy person"?
From now on, choose to identify as someone who prioritizes their health.
"I am _____ (your name) and I am someone who lives a healthy lifestyle. I eat vegetables and make the best choices possible under any given circumstances."
Changing your behavior means changing your identity—believing new things about yourself. Every action you take is a vote for the type of person you want to become.

And don't worry right now if you don't "feel" fit or healthy—it doesn't matter. You are now identifying as a healthy person.

Call it the Cher Horowitz or the "as if" method *(yes, I identify as someone who references 90s films a lot)*. Act "as if" you are already there. Keep chasing and living the behaviors that are congruent with who you identify as.

Your Personal Health Mission Statement

Having a personal health mission statement will help solidify your identity as a healthy person. Being able to fully articulate your values as someone who is constantly striving for better health reinforces this message. Here's mine as an example:

"I aim to be as healthy as I possibly can be.

I want my heart and my body to be strong so that I can do the things I love for many years to come.

It is important to me to be able to enjoy playing sports, running, hiking, skiing and practicing martial arts.

I wish to continue to hike to the summit of mountains and take in some of the most breathtaking views imaginable.

I want to be able to play with my children and role model active living and healthy eating to them, so that I may lay a foundation of healthy habits that they will hopefully carry with them as they grow into teenagers and adults.

I want to defy my own expectations as I reach my third stage of life—continuing to improve, and to avoid injuries and preventable diseases.

I want to be able to one day play active games and sports with my grandchildren—should I be blessed to have them. I want to be able to serve others around me for as long as humanly possible."

GOAL SETTING PART 2: PROCESS GOALS

When looking at your health and fat loss goals, it's absolutely critical to look past the outcome goals (i.e. lose 20 lbs, 3 dress sizes, etc) and look at the habit goals—the goals behind the outcome goals. These goals are the building blocks that form the foundation of your actions that beget your physical/body composition goals.

Goals are simply wish lists and don't transfer into anything tangible for the most part. James Clear, in his book *Atomic Habits*, does a particularly great job when he points out a few problems he has with traditional "goals." Namely:

1. **Winners and losers both have the same goals:**
   There's nothing about simply having goals that makes someone more likely to follow through than someone else with the same goals.
2. **Achieving a goal is only a temporary situation and can derail long-term progress:**
   Conquering a goal only changes things momentarily. Coaches know all too well that achieving a weight loss goal initially is only the first step and weight can easily be put back on.

Goals are transient by design. A goal-focused mindset can cause a yo-yo effect since once people achieve a goal they may revert to a previous way of living that was suboptimal. James Clear summarizes this nicely when he says, "The purpose of setting goals is to win the game. The purpose of building systems is to continue playing the game."

3. Goals can disrupt happiness:

There is an inherent assumption that our lives will be monumentally better once we achieve a goal. It creates a dichotomy as we attach happiness to an achievement—experiencing the highs if we reach it and disappointment when we don't. Attaching to outcome goals sets us up for a potential rollercoaster of emotions when what we really need is even-headedness and equanimity.

Here's an example of how to break down a goal into processes—working backwards from the outcome goal:

Outcome goal: Losing 20lbs.

Requirements: Healthier eating and more activity.

Requirements for eating healthier and being more active: Consistent food preparation and execution.

Requirements for good food preparation: A good rhythm of grocery shopping and time to prepare food.

Requirements for being more active: Creating time for intentional movement and gym access.

Requirements to create more time for food prep and activity:
-Prioritize as an important activity
-Manage time better

Requirements for better time management:
-Spend less time on tasks that do not support my health and wellness goals.
-Wake up earlier and go to sleep earlier.

Start at the bottom. What is the first process you will need for the other processes to fall into place? Put your energy into those goals and you will soon see a domino effect manifesting into physical transformation.

GOAL SETTING PART 3: THE LENS OF DISCOMFORT

Instead of asking, "What are my goals?" instead ask, "What pain am I willing to go through?"

I'll never forget the first time I read this from prominent author Mark Manson. Far too often we see goals through rose-colored glasses—picturing a utopian world where we see no obstacles.

This isn't real life, however, and we won't feel the same gusto on April 15th as we do on January 1st.

What sacrifices, discomforts or trade-offs are you willing to make to reach your goals? It is almost always best to look at goals with a realistic viewpoint of the obstacles you'll likely encounter. This will mentally prepare you for the work, rather than keep you grounded in wish lists and sure-to-dwindle enthusiasm. Enthusiasm and goal setting is fine, but there needs to be a foundation of reality and foresight of the discomfort and sacrifice it will take to reach your weight loss and health goals.

List 5 ways that you are willing to kick yourself in the comfort zone. This could be:
- Going to the bar less often, or having fewer drinks when you're out. Or both.
- Watching less TV
- Going to the gym even when you're exhausted or there is a more tempting offer.
- Getting out of bed early when all you want is more sleep.
- Cooking from scratch and spending time cutting vegetables.

Some of these activities will be a kick to your comfort zone. Some will force you to look at the obstacles you will have to face. In Day 33, I refer to researcher Gabriele Oettengen's work and her science that smacks the concept of "dreaming/law of attraction" when it comes to goal attainment. What Oettengen recommends instead is a technique she calls "mental contrasting"—basically seeing both the possibilities and obstacles to goal attainment. Balancing both the levity with gravity—seeing the reality of your obstacles. This allows just the right amount of fantasy—which can give a clear and vivid picture of your goals, and the mental clarity of the process. We will dive deeper into this in a bit.

YOUR GOAL SETTING MASTERY BLUEPRINT

It is now time to put these goals into action! We're going to do this the right way—in a way that sparks action and brings everything to life. We're about to do some deep work here so saddle up, focus and let's jump right in.

One of the most effective methods of goal setting I've seen I learned from sales/productivity/time management (and yes goal-setting) expert Brian Tracy. Tracy has written several bestsellers in the domains of entrepreneurship, sales and personal development. I will be drawing from some of his wisdom here—combining what I believe to be the most important components of action-oriented goal setting.

STEP 1: THE OUTCOME GOAL

Specific: What are the specific outcomes you want to achieve?
Measurable (and subjective): What metrics will you use? What do your subjective goals look like?
Time-oriented: What is your time frame for achieving these goals?

STEP 2: THE DEEPER DIVE

Deep why: What is your "why?" What are the most profound reasons behind your health intentions?
Process-oriented goals: What are the habit-based goals that will beget the outcome goals?
Resource-deployment: What knowledge/skills/people you will need to help you achieve your goals?
Obstacle-conscious: What are the obstacles that are standing in your way? (Pick 3-5).
Solutions-driven: What are some of the solutions to these obstacles?
Mindstorming: List 10-20 reasons why you will succeed with your goals.

Here's an example of a goal-setting worksheet. Feel free to copy as many elements of this that resonate with you, but be sure to put your own personal stamp on things.

1. Specific, measurable, time-oriented goal: *I am going to lose 25 lbs and/or 8% body fat within 6 months.*
2. Deep why: *Because I have a young family and it is important to me that I be healthy for them and be a positive role model for healthy behaviors.*
3. Process-oriented goals: *Grocery shopping 2-3x per week, food preparation on Sunday, consistent bedtime, wake up 30 min earlier, get to the gym 3x per week, get more daily steps, log food intake.*

4. Resource deployments: *I will need to work on cooking skills, exercise technique, basics of calorie counting. I will need support from my significant other to help with healthy meal prep and to look after children while I go to the gym. Being part of an online accountability group would also be helpful, as will hiring a coach.*

5. Obstacles: *Unpredictable work schedule, fatigue, waning motivation, travel schedule.*

6. Solutions: *Prioritize food prep and going to grocery stores and eating out consciously when things get busy. Prioritize sleep, use health food delivery service when needed*

7. Mindstorming: *I will lose 25 lbs and 8% body fat within 6 months by;*

1. Tracking my calories and macronutrients in My Fitness Pal

2. Getting to the gym 3-4 times per week

3. Eating out less

4. Shopping and cooking from home more

5. Hanging out more with people who do healthy things

6. Meditating/praying/practicing mindfulness

7. Getting 2000 more steps each day

8. Playing more active games with the kids

9. Riding a stationary bike while watching tv

10. Taking a bag of carrots to work daily

11. Learning 3 new healthy recipes

12. Joining a hiking group

13. Joining a support community on Facebook

14. Spending less time watching TV and surfing the smartphone

15. Hiring a coach

A variation of the above draws on the "as if" method (that is, acting as if it's already been achieved. This is an exercise called "Next Year's Christmas card" I learned from Laura Vanderkam—a time management expert in one of her TED talks. If it's less than 7 or 8 months until Christmas, use the following year's Christmas as a reference point.

We've all received those obnoxious… errrr…adorable holiday letters from friends or family —the ones that recap the year that was, the triumphs of little Luke's "mathlete" silver medal and Madeleine's goal-scoring prowess on the soccer pitch. What you are going to do is write a hypothetical letter.

Start by telling your family and friends of all your accomplishments over the year. You will tell them that you lost 25 lbs and how you have more energy, can run several miles at a time and can squat your body weight for 10 repetitions.

Next paragraph you will tell them how you succeeded. You will go into details about food logging, getting up early, forcing yourself to the gym, increasing your vegetable intake and running on the field during your child's soccer practice.

You will tell them you had lapses, stalls and moments of frustration but you persevered through them. You will tell them how your small, incremental steps built healthy habits and how you didn't follow some fad diet or cleanse but rather found a way to eat healthier and eat less. You will tell them how you found a way to get better sleep and although you spent more time at the gym, you prioritized family time.

Signed,
You.

STEP 3: BOX, LOCKS AND STACKS

Here we go—final stages of the action plan. This is where we get super specific. We have all the raw material now to build that bridge between where you are, and where you want to be. Now we execute—consistently. You are going to use time boxing, habit locks and implementation intentions (Day 41) weekly and daily to hit the process goals. These don't have to be perfect, but you must establish a stronghold of core habits and put them on repeat for this to work. Here's what this might look like. (I highly encourage customizing this to your own circumstances).

Weekly Locks

These are habits to lock into on a weekly (or multiple times weekly) basis.

PROCESS GOALS	IMPLEMENTATION INTENTIONS
Grocery Shopping (2x)	-Sunday, 8:30am at local grocery chain. -Wednesday on the way home from work, produce stand. -Pick 2 recipes and create list to shop from.
Meal Preparation (2-3x)	-Sunday: Chop and marinate tofu for the stir-fry. Cut up veggies, cook quinoa. Pack them in containers. -Wednesday: Cook chicken in oven, put in containers with lettuce and veggies.
Gym (4x)	-Sunday 11am, Monday 7pm, Wednesday, 6:15am, Thursday 6:15am. -Lower body workout on Sunday & Wednesday Upper body workout on Monday & Thursday. Hard cardio on upper body days.
Kickboxing (1x)	-Tuesday 7:30 pm at the dojo.

These are some habits to partake in daily (or at least most days). I've added a column for habit stacking as this can help increase compliance. The following are the "big rocks" of habit change and body transformation. These are as close to sacred as you can get but you may have other ideas and priorities (which is perfectly fine).

PROCESS GOAL	IMPLEMENTATION INTENTION	STACK WITH
Sleep: To bed 30 min earlier, wake up 15 min earlier.	Go to bed each night at 10pm, wake up at 6am	Reading before bed, a relaxation ritual
Pack food	Before leaving for work, pack 2-5 healthy snacks such as a can of tuna, apple, sliced peppers and a handful of almonds. Pack leftovers from dinner already packed in the to go container.	Coffee brewing, listening to morning news
Weigh in	Weigh in Monday through Friday morning.	Coffee brewing, listening to morning news
Intentional movement	Walk at lunch and after dinner	Listen to a podcast, or upbeat music playlist.
Mindfulness/meditation	Daily for 10 minutes upon waking and/or before bed using a mindfulness app.	Making bed, before sleep.

5 habits, 5 Minutes

Here's what a sample of time boxing some daily habits can look. It may seem like adopting new habits is time-consuming but it doesn't have to be. Here's a sample of some small, 5-minute blocks that can have a profound impact on your health and wellness goals.

- Meditation/mindfulness session
- Packing food into a bag or cooler
- A mobility/yoga circuit
- Body weight strength circuit (pick 5 exercises such as squats, band pulls, pushups, lunges, planks. 45 sec on, 15 seconds off).
- Food logging

The combined time to accomplish all those things is less than 30 min. Of course there are aspects of your health journey that will take longer (going to the gym and navigating a busy grocery store, to name a couple) but even picking 2-3 out of 5 of those can have a tremendous impact on your health.

Also feel free to put other non-health habits into your daily rotation. After all, you have other hobbies and interests *(at least you should)*. To give a personal example, here's a typical 5 in 5 that serves my goals of health and fitness, my business and my intellectual outlets.

- Food packing
- Mobility circuit
- Duolingo (learning Spanish)
- Quick grocery shop on route to, or on the way home from work or while out for other reasons.
- Skin care (before bed)

Putting it all Together: Prioritizing, but Keeping things Flexible

You might be thinking,

"Ok awesome, Mike, but I have family, work, elderly parents to mind and sometimes want to do something social. How do you make this work?

or

"Yeah this all sounds great, Mike but I live a busy, unpredictable life that changes all the time. I can't possibly follow something like this."

If this whole "change your life" thing seems overwhelming, don't worry, I understand. I've just thrown a lot of information at you. This won't be a perfect process, so slow down, breathe, look at yourself and your situation from in a mindful way and dive back in. Let's look at this in terms of what you CAN do. What are 1 or 2 key habits that you feel you can take on consistently? How do you feel you can get the healthiest food possible into your body and get the most intentional movement? And when all else fails and you're feeling paralyzed, refer to ANY of the days. Pick one and tackle that one directive.

The visible and invisible forces of resistance that have previously eaten away at your attempts to better your life no longer have any power. They will always be there but you will continue to grow stronger.

This will be a trial and error process that will have sticking points. There's ALWAYS a workaround, however as you are a person who strives for health, you will find a way. Make family time an active one, get the children to help grocery shop by picking their own healthy snacks. Hire babysitters, bond over a healthy meal with your spouse, get outside and run. You will go through holding patterns, internal battles, life struggles and all the rest of the junk life can throw your way. Fight for and find some predictability in your unpredictable world. Control what you can control.

What the Heck Do I Eat?

While this book is about the inner workings of change, I don't want to leave you dangling when it comes to nutrition. I'm going to make this as mercifully simple as humanly possible and I recommend you do the same. Remember the following:

All diets work (or don't):

There is no one superior way of eating for fat loss and health for everyone. Your way of eating should be specific to your goals and food preferences. The best diet is the one that gets you into a consistent caloric deficit in the least soul-sucking way possible. It should be mostly minimally processed, whole foods and contain a variety of vegetables, fruits, protein sources, good fats, beans, seeds and some fiber-rich carbohydrates.

To the above, calories matter most when it comes to weight regulation. No matter how hard pop diet book culture tries to tell you otherwise, this is a physiological reality. Eating a nutrient-dense diet with adequate protein will help you eat less overall. One affects the other and vice versa.

How many calories should I consume?

There are various online calculators and apps you can use to determine your calorie targets for fat loss. Here's one of the simplest formulas:

(10 x your weight in kilograms) + (6.25 x your height in centimeters) - (5 x your age in years) - 161.

For example, a 45-year-old woman who is 81 kilos and 165 centimeters tall would calculate her calorie consumption as:

810 (weight) + 1031 (height) - 225 (years) - 161 = 1455 calories/day to achieve fat loss

For example, a 53-year-old man who is 75 kilos and 175 centimeters tall would calculate his calorie consumption as:

700 (weight) + 1094 (height) - 265 (years) - 161 = 1368 calories/day to achieve fat loss

Strategies for Boosting Vegetable and Protein Intake

Having examined many food logs over the years I can tell you the two biggest shortcomings I see are in the vegetable and protein categories. Start there.

Vegetables

Consuming veggies isn't just a problem for children. While most grown-ups won't whine or throw them on the floor (most, not all), adult's vegetable consumption is pretty abysmal. While there are no universal guidelines for all, it's safe to say that just about everyone would benefit from a few extra servings of veggies per day.

On a per calorie basis, most veggies have the highest density of nutrients and the most disease-fighting properties. While they don't directly impact fat loss, including more of them helps push other foods out of the diet.

Here are some of the best ways to add veggies to your diet:

- Consume a vegetable at every meal (or at least most meals—I don't blame you if you don't want broccoli for breakfast)
- At dinner–make at least ½ your plate veggies. Really load up on them at dinner time (colorful and otherwise leafy vegetables with light oil/butter - not mounds of mashed potatoes loaded with butter)
- Snack on raw veggies such as; baby carrots, sliced peppers, cucumbers, broccoli and cauliflower.
- Try to build a salad every day. Use romaine lettuce or mixed greens with generous amounts of veggies.
- Add plenty of veggies to soups, stir-fries and stews.
- Try a veggie smoothie! Add some frozen or raw veggies to a fruit-based smoothie.
- Consider a greens supplement. There are several on the market. You can add them to a regular smoothie.

Ultimately aim for 3-5 servings of veggies per day. Start small, bumping your portions by 1-2 per day on average. Get used to making salads, chopping and snacking on veggies. Keep them front and center on your grocery shopping list and front and center in your fridge.

Protein

Eating adequate protein is crucial to helping you get into a calorie deficit and retain lean tissue while in that deficit. In fact, many studies have shown that boosting protein intake (in a calorie deficit) produces greater weight loss, fat mass loss, and preservation of lean mass. Also noteworthy are reductions in triglycerides, blood pressure, and waist circumference.

How much protein? I find the easiest way to calculate a good protein target is 1g per pound of your target body weight. For example if your target body weight is 150lbs, shoot for 150g/day. If you find this difficult to hit, go for at least 100g.

Here is an on-the-go list of higher protein foods for meals or snacks:

- Lettuce Roll-ups -- Roll luncheon meat, egg salad, tuna or other filling and veggies in lettuce leaves
- Lunch Meat Roll-ups -- Roll cheese or veggies in lunch meat
- Celery with tuna salad
- Hard boiled eggs
- Berries with cottage cheese
- Mini cans or packets of flavored tuna
- Jerky (beef, turkey, salmon, soy)

- Protein shake (invest in a shaker cup)
- Dried chickpeas
- Dried edamame
- Nuts/Trail mix (go light on these as they are higher in calories)

Here are a few solid ways of achieving the 100g+ mark for protein:

Example 1:
¾ cup Greek yogurt with fruit: 17g
Tuna salad (120g can): 22g
Protein shake (~1-2 scoops of whey): ~40g
Chicken stir fry (with 1 4oz chicken breast): 28g
Total Protein: 107g

Example 2:
Oatmeal with berries and a scoop of whey protein: 25g
Turkey wrap (3oz of turkey) ¼ cup low fat mozzarella cheese: 27g
Low sugar protein bar: 20g
Grilled steak salad (5oz of beef): 35g
Total Protein: 107g

Example 3:
3 eggs (whole): 18g
Cottage cheese – 1% (3/4 cup): 21g
Beef jerky (100g): 33g
Salmon (5oz): 28g
Total protein: 100g

Example 4 (Plant based):
Tofu scramble with tempeh (8oz tofu, 5 pieces of tempeh) 40g
Lentils (3oz): 18g
Whole wheat pasta with chickpeas and hemp hearts: 29g
Vegan protein shake: 15g
Total Protein: 102g

When it comes to figuring out the whole eating thing, be patient with yourself but also be doggedly persistent. Focus on one eating habit at a time and build from there. Put as many systems into place as you possibly can to encourage healthy consumption. Control the controllables with fierce consistency and exert as much control on the less-controllables as you possibly can. Stay mindful, stay big picture focused and stay in the zone of mostly good decisions.

With everything you've read to this point, I have a ton of confidence in your ability to absolutely smash your health goals. While this book isn't about the "X's and O's" of intake and exercise, I will offer some framework from which to apply what you've learned. Here is a list of what I believe to be the most important habits of health.

1. Manage sleep. Focus on getting consistently adequate and quality sleep.
2. Get some protein at every eating occasion.
3. Eat some vegetables: as many as possible.
4. Drink as much water as you can throughout the day.
5. Eat a variety of colorful, nutrient dense, fiber rich, healthy fat foods and enjoy the occasional indulgence.
6. Lift something heavy 3 times a week (twice minimum). Include Squat/lunge variations, hinging, pulling, pushing, locomotive and throw in some core work.
7. Move with intent: Move deliberately in a way that gets your heart rate up and makes you incapable of conversation.
8. Manage stress: This means not only working on constructive stress relief methods but also reframing how you view stress. Think about stress as something to embrace, roll with and learn from.
9. Nurture your relationships. Your social connections are incredibly important. Make time for the people and experiences that matter.
10. Have some fun with this. You are taking your health seriously and that's a great thing, but for goodness sake relax into it and seek out the joy and fun in everything you do.

Some Final Thoughts

I am excited for you. THRILLED actually. There is nothing that inspires me more as a coach than people taking intentional steps to change their lives. I want to thank you for making this book part of your journey. I sincerely hope that some of what I have said has resonated with you so that you may move forward in your health quest. Know you are capable and know that you deserve 100% of the credit for your results. YOU are the one putting the work in, showing up daily and fighting life's daily battles.

I've laid out templates, ideas and strategies but when you put this book down, I will have not given you the fish, I will have taught you HOW to fish. You are now equipped with a bulletproof mindset, the ability to implement simple yet effective strategies through shaping your environment and action-orientation.

The concepts may take some time to sink in and I advise referring back to the principles as often as necessary. Most importantly, just get out there and take charge of your weight loss and your physical, mental, emotional and spiritual health.

Someone once told me that life can be seen as a juggling act—each ball representing an aspect of life. Some of these balls are made of rubber and include things like TV, movies, YouTube, social media consumption, unpaid extra work, friends who are energy vampires, committees that you aren't passionate about.

Other balls are made of crystal and include family, friends, career, faith and yes, health. When we juggle through life it's important to keep those crystal balls sacred—safe from falling. The ones made of rubber aren't important—let them fall. Put your energy fully into the crystal balls.

Your family, friends, work life and spiritual life all benefit when you prioritize your health. And guess what? You may very well become a role model for someone else who might need a little bit of a spark. Imagine how many lives you can impact through your personal steps of growth. The chances of you being born are approximately 1 in 400 TRILLION. You are meant to do something special. You are meant to get out there and live a life of health and joy.

The visible and invisible forces of resistance will still try and pull you away from what matters. This time is different, however. This time you are prepared, equipped with the right mindset, the crucial habits and your personal action plan. Your why and your identity are way bigger than your obstacles. You have made a conscious choice to be in control of your health destiny. You are now free of the reasons why you can't do this and this time you will NOT ring that bell.

You are meant to be healthy and you deserve the best chance at being healthy. This is your time, this is your moment. Take it and run with it—without looking back.

I'm here for you—cheering you on, encouraging you and empowering you to push yourself past your perceived limitations. Reach out to me and let me know how you're doing. I'm here to help.

Mike

APPENDIX

While technology can certainly detract from your goals in many ways, we can also use it to leverage your progress.

Here are some apps that I've found to be helpful in grooving excellent health habits. I find there are 3 helpful categories of apps that are especially helpful.

1. Tracking.
2. Habit Tracking and
3. Productivity/Smartphone limiting.

Calorie/Macronutrient Tracking Apps:

MyFitnessPal

Lose It

MyMacros+

Habit Tracking Apps:

Nudge Coach

Habitica

StiKK

Productivity Apps:

Offtime

Moment

Flipd

Still Need Help?

Lean Minded offers a comprehensive program with 6 Modules, meal plan templates, videos and access to a private facebook group.

I also take one-on-one coaching clients on a limited basis. Visit www.leanminded.com for more details.

First Paperback Edition: November, 2019

ISBN: 978-0-9936759-1-1

Edited by Donna Barker
Book and Cover Design by Sophia Ellis

CPSIA information can be obtained
at www.ICGtesting.com
Printed in the USA
LVHW071144151219
640578LV00003B/42/P